LECTURE NOTES ON
MEDICINE IN GENERAL PRACTICE

Life is fired at us at point blank range.
We cannot say, 'Wait till I have
sorted things out'.

Ortega y Gasset

LECTURE NOTES ON MEDICINE IN GENERAL PRACTICE

CONRAD M. HARRIS

MEd, MB, ChB, FRCGP, DRCOG

Senior Lecturer
Department of General Practice
St Mary's Hospital Medical School, London

SECOND EDITION

Blackwell Scientific Publications
OXFORD   LONDON   EDINBURGH
BOSTON   PALO ALTO   MELBOURNE

First published 1980
Reprinted 1981
Second edition 1984

Set by DMB (Typesetting)
Oxford
Printed and bound by
Billing & Sons Ltd
Worcester

DISTRIBUTORS

USA
  Blackwell Mosby Book Distributors
  11830 Westline Industrial Drive
  St Louis, Missouri 63141

Canada
  Blackwell Mosby Book Distributors
  120 Melford Drive, Scarborough
  Ontario M1B 2X4

Australia
  Blackwell Scientific Book Distributors
  31 Advantage Road, Highett
  Victoria 3190

British Library
Cataloguing in Publication Data

Harris, Conrad M.
  Lecture notes on medicine in general
  practice.
  1. Family medicine
  I. Title
  362.1'72   R729.5.G4

  ISBN 0-632-00604-8

Contents

List of tables

Preface to the First Edition

This book is written for medical students. Its content keeps within the bounds of basic medical education. It starts with a section on morbidity, because diagnosis is a concept familiar to the student, even if what is diagnosed in general practice is not always so familiar. Psychosocial aspects of clinical work in this setting are considered next, because students find them so crucial in understanding what is going on. The section on the resources available to the doctor is to fill gaps in knowledge, while that on the skills required should give a better insight into what is observed. The final section, on the clinical roles of the general practitioner, is a summary and synthesis of all that has gone before. It offers the student a framework for organising his learning and for thinking about the future.

No attempt has been made to describe the diagnosis and management of particular illnesses, though this is the major activity of the general practitioners with whom the student works. Individual clinical problems are best discussed with the doctor concerned, using knowledge gleaned from other parts of the medical course.

For the facts and ideas used in this book I am indefinably indebted to many colleagues in academic and non-academic general practice, to a great deal of published research, and to several thousand medical students. I had many helpful comments from Paul Freeling, Brian Jarman, Bill Styles and Hugh Tunstall Pedoe on the penultimate draft, and in the practical problems of writing a book I acknowledge with gratitude the help of my secretary, Frances Hanson.

Conrad M. Harris
June 1979

Preface to the Second Edition

The opportunity has been taken to revise the text, update the statistics quoted and add material where it seemed to be necessary in the light of experience. The new section 'Notes for Students Interviewing Patients' should provide help in a particularly difficult area.

The First Edition proved useful not only to undergraduates, but also to those general practitioners who teach them in their surgeries and to vocational trainees moving into their training practices. I hope that this Second Edition will be even more so.

Conrad M. Harris

I. Morbidity in general practice

Introduction

Students sometimes say that 'real' illness is rare in general practice. 'Real' seems to imply a degree of drama or danger, pathology of the sort described in textbooks, or the applicability of some high technology: the kind of illness, in fact, which is familiar from experience in hospital. One of the reasons why medicine needs to be taught also in the setting of general practice is that there the student can learn about a wider range of illnesses and about other conditions which affect people's health.

In the chapters of this section, the morbidity seen in general practice will be considered in four ways:
1 By comparing it with hospital morbidity, in each case using information gathered nationally.
2 By looking in greater detail at the morbidity in an 'average' practice, i.e. national data scaled down to a population the size of a general practitioner's list.
3 By considering the most important reasons why practices differ from the 'average'.
4 By suggesting a way of classifying the illnesses seen that allows for different kinds of importance.

Before doing so, four warnings must be made:

Putting diagnostic labels on the problems seen in general practice is frequently difficult and sometimes impossible.

Diagnoses are liable to error because of deficiencies in what the doctor recognises, or chooses to recognise for the purposes of recording.

The data used in this section were recorded by doctors interested in collecting data; these doctors may differ from other general practitioners.

Diagnosis is an ordered summation of what is known about a patient's condition, and is used to guide the doctor's intervention:

3

this means that in general practice many non-medical factors have to be taken into account. Psychological and social considerations are always important; disease labels are never enough.

With these warnings in mind, we can look at what is known about morbidity in general practice.

1. General practice and hospital morbidity compared

One way of comparing the different patterns of morbidity seen in hospital and general practice is to make use of the International Classification of Diseases (ICD). This categorises conditions mainly by body systems, each of the categories having further divisions and subdivisions. Table 1.1 shows how morbidity is distributed in the two situations.

Moving into finer focus, we can look *within* the main ICD categories for differences. Table 1.2 takes three of them—V, VII and VIII—and compares the frequency with which some of the conditions they contain are seen. Not all categories show differences between the two settings as marked as these.

The reason for the differences between the two patterns of morbidity lies in a process of selection. A general practitioner with an average sized list will refer no more than one or two of the patients he sees each day to an outpatient department, and send only about one patient a week into hospital as an emergency admission. In teaching hospitals the patients may be especially highly selected, reflecting mainly the particular interests of the consultants in charge. The student may learn a great deal from studying the illnesses of these patients, but not much about the pattern of morbidity in the community.

Comparing diagnostic labels is useful, but it has limitations. Even when a condition is common in both hospital and general practice it may be seen in a rather different perspective in the two situations. Duodenal ulcers, for example, present dramatically in hospital, with severe exacerbation, haemorrhage, perforation or pyloric obstruction. In general practice patients are seen with their ulcers over many years, often with no symptoms, sometimes with moderate misery and only rarely with major complications. Also the very early signs and symptoms of serious disease are brought to the general practitioner at a stage when it may be difficult to distinguish them from the manifestations of illnesses that are less significant.

Table 1.1   General practice and hospital morbidity compared
by ICD heading

ICD heading		GP %	Hospital %
I	Infective and parasitic diseases	4	2
II	All neoplasms	1	8
III	Endocrine, nutritional and metabolic disease	2	2
IV	Diseases of blood and blood-forming organs	1	1
V	Mental disorders	10	4
VI	Diseases of the nervous system and sense organs	7	5
VII	Diseases of the circulatory system	8	9
VIII	Diseases of the respiratory system	19	8
IX	Diseases of the digestive system	4	10
X	Diseases of the genitourinary system	5	8
XI	Conditions of pregnancy, childbirth and the puerperium	10	19
XII	Diseases of the skin and subcutaneous tissue	6	2
XIII	Diseases of the musculoskeletal system and connective tissues	7	3
XIV	Congenital anomalies	0	2
XV	Certain causes of perinatal morbidity and mortality	0	1
XVI	Symptoms and ill-defined conditions	8	6
XVII	Accidents, poisonings and violence	5	10
XVIII	Prophylactic procedures and other medical examinations	3	0

NB   Hospital data include psychiatric illness and are based on inpatient statistics. Antenatal care data from general practice have been moved from XVIII to XI.

Table 1.2 General practice and hospital morbidity compared within three ICD headings

		GP (% of consultations)	Hospital (% of admissions)
V	*Mental disorders*		
	Psychoneuroses	60	17
	Schizophrenic and paranoid states	3	17
	Personality disorders	1	9
	Senile and presenile dementia	1	7
	Alcoholism and drug dependence	1	6
VII	*Circulatory system*		
	Hypertensive disease	31	5
	Angina and IHD	14	8
	Cerebrovascular disease	8	19
	Acute myocardial infarction	6	18
	Thrombosis and embolism	1	5
VIII	*Respiratory system*		
	Nasopharyngitis and influenza	28	<1
	Acute tonsillitis and pharyngitis	20	6
	Acute bronchitis	20	4
	Pneumonia	2	12
	Hypertrophy of tonsils and adenoids	<1	26

REFERENCE SOURCES

OPCS (1974) *Morbidity Statistics from General Practice Second National Study 1970-71.* HMSO, London.

OPCS (1973) *Report on Hospital In-patient Enquiry for 1971.* HMSO, London.

DHSS (1973) *Psychiatric Hospitals and Units in England and Wales 1971.* HMSO, London.

WHO (1977) *Manual of the International Statistical Classification of Diseases, Injuries and Causes of Death*, Ninth Revision. HMSO, London.

2. The 'average' practice

Data collected from many practices can be aggregated and then used to show what may be expected in a notional practice with 2000 patients, this now being roughly the average list size in the UK. If the original practices were carefully chosen, this notional 'average' practice will reflect characteristics of the population of the country as a whole. The National Morbidity Studies (NMS), based on recordings from a large number of practices, provide the most useful collections of figures for this exercise.

Other sources of data which can be applied to the 'average' practice are also available: the most important are the annual General Household Surveys (GHS), the decennial Census, various statistical returns published by the Department of Health and Social Security, and *ad hoc* surveys commissioned for specific purposes or arising from research studies.

For reasons which we will consider later, few practices will resemble the 'average' practice, but the concept is a useful one for giving the student an idea of what to expect—provided that he remembers that it is a tool rather than a description of something real.

In the 'average' practice, with a population of 2000 patients, we would expect:

1 Nearly 500 children under the age of 16 and about 300 people aged 65 or more (100 of them being 75 or older). About 500 married couples; 33 one-parent families; four children in the care of the Local Authority; and two adults in prison. Fifteen marriages, six divorces, 25 births and 23 deaths in the course of a year—six of the deaths taking place in the home.

2 About 7500 consultations in a year. 700 patients will not consult at all in this time, but it is customary to calculate consultation rates on the whole practice population rather than on the 1300 who are seen. Some 1200 of the consultations will take place in the patient's home and roughly 25 will be at night. Elderly patients have proportionately the greatest number of house calls. The data in Table 2.1 come from the 1981 GHS; telephone consultations are included, and these make up 7% of the total.

Table 2.1 Consultation rates for different age groups, by sex and by ratio of surgery to home consultations

Age	0-4	5-15	16-44	45-64	65-74	75+	All ages
Male	6.7	2.5	2.3	3.7	3.9	5.8	3.2
Female	5.5	2.7	4.9	4.0	4.6	6.0	4.4
Surgery: home	4.9	7.6	12.1	8.8	2.6	1.0	5.6

GHS 1981

3 In terms of some conditions with which the student is familiar, each year eight patients suffer an acute myocardial infarction, eight get pneumonia, four develop appendicitis and three take an overdose. Table 2.2 gives the frequency with which 50 common conditions will be seen. Note that they are *not* frequencies of new diagnoses.

Table 2.2 Frequency of consultation for common conditions in the 'average' practice

Frequency	Condition for consultation (alphabetical order)
>3 per week	Acute bronchitis; antenatal care; contraception; D & V; hypertension; menstrual disorders; psychoneurosis; superficial injury; tonsillitis & pharyngitis; URTI
1-3 per week	Acute back syndromes; angina and IHD; asthma; cervical smear; chronic bronchitis; congestive heart failure; conjunctivitis; eczema/dermatitis; ear wax; malignant neoplasm; obesity; osteoarthritis; otitis media; sprains and strains; UTI; vaginal discharge
1-4 per month	Acne; boils; cerebrovascular disease; constipation; diabetes; DU; dyspepsia; epilepsy; haemorrhoids; herpes zoster; insomnia; measles; migraine; myocardial infarct; otitis externa; pneumonia; rheumatoid arthritis; schizophrenia; sinusitis; thyroid disease; undiagnosed rashes; urticaria; VVs; warts

REFERENCE SOURCES

OPCS (1974) *Morbidity Statistics from General Practice. Second National Study 1970-71.* HMSO, London.
OPCS (1983) *General Household Survey 1981.* HMSO, London.

3. Why practices differ from the 'average'

There are many reasons why the morbidity seen in any real practice differs from that of the 'average' practice. The most important depend on where the practice is situated, but the characteristics of the doctors and perhaps of the other staff make some difference.

Morbidity varies from one area to another in ways which can be considered separately, though they are usually interrelated.

AGE

The age structure of a practice population will usually reflect that of the surrounding area fairly accurately. It is important for two reasons: the very young and the elderly have the highest consulting rates (see Table 2.1), and morbidity is different in different age groups (see Tables 3.1 and 3.2).

The 1981 Census shows that in East Sussex one person in four is aged 65 or over, whereas in Cleveland only about one person in nine is in this age group. Many areas have more than 7% of the population under the age of five, while Camden has only 4.5%. There will be a different emphasis in the clinical problems faced by doctors in a south-coast retirement resort, a new industrial estate with predominantly young families, and a city area populated by mobile young adults.

SOCIAL CLASS

The Registrar-General's system of classifying people into five groups by occupation is crude and in many ways out of date, but it does demonstate large disparities in the relative occurrence of many illnesses. The reasons for these disparities are often not clear, but nearly all the common causes of death and much morbidity show

11

Table 3.1 Consultation rates (per 1000 population)
for the commonest conditions of childhood

Condition	0-4	5-14	All ages
Prophylactic procedures	602	96	316
Acute nasopharyngitis	549	173	152
Acute otitis media	294	130	53
Bronchitis and bronchiolitis	272	108	112
Pharyngitis and tonsillitis	253	218	111
Diarrhoea and vomiting	212	54	66
Eczema and dermatitis	130	38	52
Cough	128	56	34
Conjunctivitis	79	21	24
Superficial injury	56	69	68
Catarrh	54	26	19
Viral warts	6	65	18
All conditions	3632	1928	3010

NMS 2

Table 3.2 Consultation rates (per 1000 population) for the
commonest conditions of the elderly

Condition	65-74	75 +	All ages
Hypertension	300	223	79
Osteoarthritis	178	301	57
Acute bronchitis and bronchiolitis	166	194	112
All neoplasms	154	149	45
Chronic bronchitis	152	132	38
Angina + IHD	136	190	35
Depressive neurosis	118	91	90
Congestive heart failure	93	301	26
Cerebrovascular disease	80	180	20
Prophylactic procedures	75	77	316
Anxiety neurosis	74	50	73
Acute nasopharyngitis	69	62	152
All conditions	3764	4475	3010

NMS 2

a gradient which favours the upper social classes. This is discussed again in Chapter 6, and detailed evidence can be found in textbooks of epidemiology. The amount of illness and the consulting rates of practices in Social Class IV-V areas are undoubtedly higher than those found in wealthy suburbs. The pattern of morbidity is also different.

REGION

Many diseases show quite large regional variation within England and Wales. One common pattern is a difference between the north and the south: for example, respiratory disease is more common in the north of England and in south Wales, than in the south of England. Some variation may be related to factors in the soil or water, e.g. stomach cancer or pernicious anaemia. The distribution of the handicapped is also uneven. In Manchester they were shown to form 5.4% of the population, compared with 0.81% in Cambridgeshire. Variations *within* one region were also dramatic: in Hackney 4.52% of the population was handicapped, compared with 2.24% in Camden. It may be difficult to demonstrate some of these differences at the level of individual practices.

CULTURE

A little of the difference between practices may be explained by traditional responses to illness in the local community: traditions in an occupation which dominates the area, or in ethnic groups, for example. One practice, with a very mixed population, has found that its Irish patients have the lowest consultation rates and its patients from the Indian sub-continent the highest.

TOWN AND COUNTRY

In general, death rates are lower in the country. This is clearly true of deaths from malignancy and respiratory disease but there is no clear pattern for circulatory disease, and male death rates from accidents are higher. Table 3.3 shows differences between general practice consulting rates in town and country which are therefore not entirely predictable.*

* Inner-city practice is greatly under-represented in the Second National Morbidity Survey from which these figures are taken.

Table 3.3 Comparative consulting rates (per 1000 population) for fifteen conditions in urban and rural practices

Condition	Urban	Rural
Acute pharyngitis and tonsillitis	119	91
Anxiety neurosis	79	56
Acute otitis media	55	50
Conjunctivitis	25	20
Hay fever	18	12
Depressive neurosis	86	102
Hypertension	73	95
Superficial injury	60	88
Osteoarthritis	53	70
All neoplasms	40	58
Angina and IHD	31	44
Congestive heart failure	23	34
Cerebrovascular disease	16	30
Diabetes	14	26
Anaemia (iron deficiency)	15	24
All	2941	3195

NMS 2

Minor infections cause more consultations in urban practice, and this may well be due to urban living conditions, but we do not really know how much of the difference is due to greater frequency of the conditions, and how much to the behaviour of the sufferers in consulting a doctor.

INDIVIDUAL CHARACTERISTICS

This is a poorly documented subject, and evidence about possible effects is mainly anecdotal. On the basis of their personalities, age, sex, and special interests, the doctors within one practice do seem to attract a particular clientele. The reputation of a practice as a whole, arising from its organisation and atmosphere as well as the activities of its medical and non-medical staff, may play a part in determining the practice population and hence the morbidity seen, but this is very difficult to measure.

REFERENCE SOURCES

OPCS (1974) *Morbidity Statistics from General Practice. Second National Study 1970-71* (NMS 2) HMSO, London.
CIPFA (1979) *Personal Social Service Statistics, 1978-79 Estimates.*

4. Which illnesses are important

We have considered the illness expected in an 'average' practice and the reasons why there is bound to be deviation from the 'average' in any individual practice. Without forgetting the limitations set by the warnings in the introduction to this section, we can see that a pattern of the morbidity of general practice has emerged; there remains the need to put it into some kind of perspective.

A traditional approach has been to classify illnesses as Minor, Major and Chronic, but this is unsatisfactory for several reasons. Distinctions are often quite arbitrary, and can be made safely only with the benefit of hindsight. There is a danger that patients as well as illnesses may be categorised in this way. It is more helpful, and certainly more stimulating, to recognise five (slightly overlapping) classes of illness, all of which are important. They correspond to the problems of medicine in general practice.

1 Illnesses that are common. The definition is arbitrary, but illnesses newly diagnosed at least once a month could be so described.

2 Illnesses that are rarer but life-threatening: myocardial infarction, strokes, severe depression, appendicitis, cancer and meningitis, for example. The aims of prevention or early diagnosis have implications both for the skills that the general practitioner requires and for the way in which his practice is organised.

3 Illnesses that are chronic and handicapping: chronic bronchitis, osteoarthritis and rheumatoid arthritis, congestive heart failure, diabetes, epilepsy, schizophrenia, parkinsonism, and multiple sclerosis, for example.

4 Illnesses for which early treatment is especially worthwhile: myxoedema, pernicious anaemia, glaucoma, and congenital dislocation of the hip, for example.

5 Illnesses that are usually minor, but serious for a vulnerable group: rubella for pregnant women, fractured ribs for chronic

15

bronchitics, chest infections for people in congestive heart failure, influenza for diabetics, and measles for children with cystic fibrosis, for example.

II. Psychosocial aspects

Introduction

Students working in general practice are immediately struck by the importance of psychosocial factors. These factors determine, in part, what symptoms people experience, how they are interpreted, and whether or not they will be presented to a doctor. They are significant in the relationship between patient and doctor, for they affect both diagnosis and management. The problems they produce are inextricably interwoven with the effects of pathological processes. In dealing with them, the general practitioner has the advantage of learning about them in the environment where they are most clearly displayed—patients' homes.

These psychosocial aspects of medicine are considered in the next five chapters.

5. Symptoms

Traditionally, patients complain of symptoms. The doctor may respond by asking himself either, 'What pathology lies behind them?' or, 'Why is this patient consulting me?' One of the distinguishing marks of general practice is that it is particularly concerned with the second question. The more skilful and discerning general practitioners are in referring their patients, the more irrelevant the second question becomes to the hospital specialist, because its answer is in the letter of referral. The proper diagnostic task of the specialist is to find the pathology behind the symptoms, and if there seems to be none in his limited field, this does not mean that there is none elsewhere. The specialist who tells a patient that there is nothing wrong with him is going outside the specialist role.

Since there is no limit to the reasons why patients consult their general practitioners, the latter cannot assume that there is any pathology to be pursued. 'Why is this patient consulting me?' is therefore always an important question, and remains so even when the pattern of the symptoms makes it likely that pathology *is* present.

HEALTH

The concept of 'health' is a difficult one. 'Good health' is sometimes defined as though it is an entity in its own right—not just the absence of any kind of illness, but the presence of some rather mysterious positive factor as well. Many authors prefer to see it as relative and subjective—describing the attitude of an individual to his circumstances even when these include obvious disability. In surveys people are often allowed to define health in their own terms.

A set of questions in the 1977 General Household Survey illustrates this well. Two-thirds of the men and half of the women said that their health in the preceding year had, on the whole, been good. They were asked both about chronic and short-term problems of

19

the previous two weeks, and clearly it was the former which influenced their opinion more.

CHRONIC HEALTH PROBLEMS

56% or the men and 70% of the women in the sample said that they had some kind of health problem all the time, or one that kept returning. Such problems were reported more by women than by men in all age groups. They increased with age for both sexes, but the rates converged in the older groups. More than two-thirds of the sufferers took some special kind of care—men being more likely to take things slowly or be careful of the weather, and women to take medication, most often something prescribed by a doctor. Of the whole population surveyed, 18% of the men and 28% of the women were taking prescribed medication all the time for chronic health problems. There were consistently more chronic problems in the lower social classes.

SHORT-TERM ILL HEALTH

The pattern of short-term problems (i.e. those which had occurred within the previous fortnight and were not apparently connected with any chronic problem) was very different. The variation by sex was less marked at all ages, though women did report more than men—57% to 52%. Episodes *decreased* with age—though possibly

Table 5.1 Health problems experienced—by assessment of own health in the preceding year and by sex; persons aged sixteen and over

Problems experienced	Own assessments of year's health (%)					
	Good		Fairly good		Not good	
	M	F	M	F	M	F
None	90	86	10	12	0	1
Short-term only (previous two weeks)	82	76	17	22	1	2
Chronic only	51	46	33	38	16	16
Short-term plus chronic	47	38	39	42	15	20
Total	65	53	26	34	9	14

GHS 1977

this might have been due to the elderly relating their acute problems to their increasingly common chronic problems.

Table 5.2 Persons reporting short-term health problems in the 14 days before interview; by age and sex

Age	Males %	Females %
16-44	56	61
45-64	49	55
65-74	44	53
75 +	45	51
Total	52	57

45% of the men and 49% of the women took some kind of medication for a short-term problem in the two weeks, but except in the elderly this medication was usually not prescribed by a doctor. Short-term health problems did not vary significantly across the social classes.

SYMPTOMS AND HEALTH

An earlier, smaller survey found that about two-thirds of the population regarded their health as excellent or good, about one-fifth as fair, and about one-tenth as poor. Almost everyone experienced symptoms—in two weeks, adults on average had 3.9 symptoms; those who described their health as excellent or good had 2.5, while those who thought it poor had 6.2. Excellent health went with 'no symptoms' in 4% of the population; poor or fair health went with 'no symptoms' in less than 1%.

The symptoms of the healthy were different from those of the unhealthy: the former were more likely to have headaches, skin troubles, accidents and trouble with teeth or feet; the latter to suffer from breathlessness, faintness, loss of appetite, undue tiredness or a raised temperature. Some symptoms were thus taken more seriously than others.

THE COMMONEST SYMPTOMS

No one knows for certain which symptoms are the commonest, but the largest survey among United Kingdom adults suggests the following order: respiratory, circulatory, ill-defined, due to accidents, digestive, musculoskeletal, those affecting the CNS and sense organs, and mental. Note that these symptoms were interpreted to fit a medical classification. Other surveys have given similar results, though with some variations in the order. Mental symptoms usually come higher in the list.

DISTRIBUTION OF SYMPTOMS

Symptoms are not distributed evenly in the population.

AGE

As they get older, people are less likely to describe their health as excellent, but the number of symptoms they report does not increase in the way that might be expected. Perhaps the elderly ascribe some to their age, or possibly they concentrate on those that are most severe. They are more likely to experience breathlessness, indigestion, insomnia, constipation, musculoskeletal pains and faintness, while younger adults have headaches, sore throats, bad nerves, rashes, accidents and dental troubles. Children are more likely than adults to suffer the effects of accidents, tooth and gum troubles and vomiting; younger children have more symptoms than older children.

SEX

Girls and boys have an equal number of symptoms, but women have more than men—especially constipation, nervous symptoms and weight problems. Men are more likely to have upper respiratory symptoms.

SOCIAL CLASS

Digestive complaints seem to be commonest in Social Classes I and II, and musculoskeletal symptoms in Classes IV and V. The higher social classes apparently experience fewer symptoms.

MARITAL STATUS

The unmarried report most digestive symptoms; the widowed,

separated and divorced most of every kind of mental symptom except headache, which is commonest in the married.

OTHER

People of an anxious disposition experience more symptoms than others. Many kinds of symptoms are commoner in the unemployed than in those with a job.

SYMPTOMS PRESENTED TO THE DOCTOR

Probably no more than a quarter of the illnesses in the population are taken to the doctor. In one group of women aged 20-44 (a group with a high consulting rate) only one symptom in 38 resulted in a medical consultation. Symptoms are often ignored, and self-medication is very common—as many as two-thirds of all adults are likely to take non-prescribed preparations in a period of two weeks.

People assess their symptoms according to their knowledge, expectations and fears, and get advice from others before they decide to go to the doctor. In the women mentioned above, 5% of sore throats but only 0.5% of headaches resulted in a consultation. One practice found that impairment of hearing was commonest in people over 65, though consultations about deafness were most frequent in patients between 45 and 64.

Age, sex, social class, marital status and employment status all play some part in determining consultation, and immigrant groups may differ from the native population in their reactions. Indians appear unduly alarmed by 'fever' to British doctors who have not considered how serious it might be in India.

There are broad social trends which have no clear explanation: people declare themselves sick more frequently than they did 10-15 years ago, and they stay off work longer.

INTERPRETING THE SYMPTOMS

The probabilities on which standard differential diagnoses are based were established for populations of referred patients; they may not be very helpful in general practice. For example, haemoptysis is said by medical teachers to be a serious presenting symptom, but it rarely turns out to be of serious import in this country now. Vertigo suggests different probabilities in general practice from those that would be accepted in an ENT clinic—a study found that no diagnosis could be made or that the cause was emotional in more than half the patients who presented with it. Chest pain is very much more likely to have an emotional cause than to be due to coronary artery disease.

Sometimes the doctor finds a patient's behaviour more remarkable than his symptoms—usually when there is more distress than seems warranted. The cause may be fears about the meaning of the symptoms, or about something quite different—the use of symptoms as a so-called 'passport' into the surgery (see Chapters 7 and 9).

More confusing still are the occasions when the doctor agrees with the patient's own assessment of a minor condition like a cold, but can detect no undue distress to account for the consultation. The explanation may lie in behaviour learned by the patient as a child—in his family a cold may have been a good reason to go to the doctor, and he continues the tradition naturally in his adult life.

Not infrequently the general practitioner responds directly to the symptoms without making a diagnosis. It may be clear that one patient needs urgent admission to hospital, or that no action is required for another, long before the doctor has determined precisely what is wrong.

REFERENCE SOURCES

OPCS (1973 and 1979) *General Household Surveys, 1971 and 1977.* HMSO, London.

Wadsworth M.E.J., Butterfield W.J.H. & Blaney R. (1971) *Health and Sickness : the Choice of Treatment.* Tavistock, London.

Morrell D.C. (1976) *An Introduction to Primary Care.* Churchill Livingstone, Edinburgh.

6. Social factors and social problems

An epidemiology course may be the most appropriate time for the students to learn how the experience of illness is related to social class, but a course in general practice has no equal for learning in two other areas: the importance of the particular social context in which an illness occurs, and the close relationship of medical with social problems. All three topics are important.

ILLNESS AND SOCIAL CLASS

Social class is a complicated and contentious topic, but for the purposes of this book it means no more than grouping people into categories on the basis of occupation. The simpler systems have many anomalies; they are still used because they continue to offer a powerful and useful tool in social analysis. The most widely known is the classification adopted in the 1971 Census. The experiences of life of members of these classes differ in many ways that concern doctors. The term 'gradient' is used to describe differences which change in a consistent way between Classes I and V. Evidence of such gradients in relation to birth, death, illness and use of health services is easy to find; a few examples follow.

BIRTH

Survival at birth is related to length of gestation which is most likely to be normal in Class I (80%) and least likely in Class V (66%). Stillbirth and post-neonatal death rates also show marked class gradients in favour of Class I.

DEATH

Life expectancy and age at death are class-related; in all age groups

Table 6.1 Typical occupations in the Registrar-General's social classification

Social class	Typical occupations	% of population
I	*Professional*: doctors, lawyers, university lecturers	4
II	*Intermediate*: nurses, chiropodists, MPs, teachers	18
III	*Skilled*: (non manual) secretaries, draughtsmen (manual) bus drivers, butchers, carpenters	49 $\begin{cases} 21 \\ 28 \end{cases}$
IV	*Semi-skilled*: barmen, bus conductors, postmen	21
V	*Unskilled*: labourers, office cleaners, stevedores	8

the mean annual death-rate increases from Class I to Class V. Maternal mortality is more than three times as high in Class V as in Class I, and all the commoner causes of death (except breast cancer) have gradients favouring Class I.

ILLNESS

Class V has the highest proportion of families where adverse circumstances like low income, bad housing, and poor education affect the children's health. Bedwetting, squint, stuttering, dental disease, fits, bronchitis, pneumonia and infective diarrhoea, for example, are more frequent; children are shorter and more often have unintelligible speech. Comparing women with a child under the age of six, one study found psychiatric disturbance (usually depression) to be nearly eight times more common in the working-class (31%) than the middle-class group (4%).

In adults, differences between the classes appear both for acute and chronic illnesses, though they are much more marked in the latter. The excess morbidity in Class V seems to occur in the younger adults.

USE OF HEALTH SERVICES

People in the lower social classes on the whole consult their general practitioners more often, though for infants the gradient goes the opposite way, and for the elderly class differences largely disappear.

On the other hand, medical need is greater in Classes IV and V, and it is possible to show that Classes I and II consult more frequently relative to the amount of illness they perceive themselves as suffering. Middle-class consultations last longer; they have a greater clinical content, where working-class consultations have a greater administrative content. Working-class people tend to have doctors with larger lists, and one survey showed Classes I and II to be making more use of the resources of the 'primary care team' as a whole, including, for instance, the services of the health visitor. Referral for specialist care is more than twice as likely for Social Class I as for Class V patients, and the familiar gradient also appears in preventive medicine—in immunisation and visits to the dentist for example. The percentage of men who smoke is twice as great in Class V as in Class I.

Exactly which factors—genetic, environmental, or cultural—in the lives of people from the lower social classes cause particular illnesses is unknown, and elucidating them is one of the major challenges facing medicine. Another challenge is the matching of medical resources to medical need. The Inverse Care Law described by one general practitioner puts the position clearly, 'The availability of good medical care tends to vary inversely with the need of the population served' (Tudor Hart).

Students attached to practices whose patients come from all social classes have a chance to see how articulate, middle-class patients expect more, and make better use of, medical services than do the rest of the population, and how doctors may respond differently to the differing approaches, expectations and demands of patients from various strata of society.

ILLNESSES AND THEIR SOCIAL CONTEXT

In general practice it is easy to appreciate how a patient's illness and social circumstances are related, because the social circumstances are visible. Reporting the histories they have prepared, students automatically describe the patient's background: without it the reports would seem unnatural and lose their point. It is also obvious how any medical intervention has consequences for the patient's social roles. This is quite separate from the idea that some illnesses have a social component in their aetiology. The point is that *no* illness can be understood or managed without reference to the unique circumstances of the patient who suffers it.

The importance of the social context applies in hospital too—in outpatient therapy and in the timing of admission to the ward or discharge from it, for example. There are two differences in hospital: first, the conditions treated more often present the sort of immediate threat that justifies the overriding of some social considerations; and secondly, the social context is not so visible. In general practice the student can learn by direct observation about an aspect of practice which is important to all clinicians.

For any kind of doctor planning the management of a man with diabetes, it is as necessary to know that the patient has a good income and a competent, caring wife as it is to discover that he has neither. Any kind of doctor who recommends rest, exercise, twice weekly visits to the physiotherapy department, or greater intimacy with a spouse will lose credibility, and therefore the power to help, if his advice does not fit the circumstances of the patient to whom he gives it. This may seem too obvious to need emphasis, but doctors do forget it. *All diagnoses have a social component, whether or not there are social problems.* This is one of the more important lessons to take from the course in general practice.

ILLNESS AND SOCIAL PROBLEMS

A simple view of illness and social problems is that either can 'cause' the other. For example:

ILLNESS 'CAUSING' SOCIAL PROBLEMS

An active woman of 62, living alone, has a stroke. She recovers most of her bodily functions, but feels unsteady and unable to go out. Her only daughter lives in Australia.

A widower of 30, with two children, has a prolapsed intervertebral disc. He spends a fortnight in bed, with some help from a neighbour, but less strictly than the doctor advises. He then has to go into hospital and laminectomy seems likely.

SOCIAL PROBLEMS 'CAUSING' ILLNESS

An old man, lonely after his wife's death, and living in poor circumstances, develops hypothermia the following winter.

A young woman, with a husband who drinks heavily and who is struggling to look after three children and an invalid mother, injures her baby. She has an acute emotional breakdown for which she is admitted to hospital.

To generalise:

a Wherever there is chronic illness there are likely to be social problems, and whenever a new illness develops in someone who has little support, a social problem can arise.

b Illness 'caused' by social problems is largely a matter of medical definition. Until hypothermia was recognised, the old man would have been thought of merely as cold; emotional states were always known to have social repercussions, but when called psychiatric illnesses they enter the doctor's province.

In real life the idea of cause and effect here is unhelpful; illness and social problems merge into each other. The two histories which follow were reported by students who had just completed their course in general practice.

The Rileys. Mrs Riley, a woman in her middle twenties, brought her six-month-old baby to the doctor and complained that he kept screaming during the night. The doctor found nothing physically wrong except that the baby was very overweight. Mrs Riley was a fat Finnish woman, married to an Irishman. It seemed that her husband was shouting at her because he could not get to sleep and had to be up at half past six. They were living in one room and were to be thrown out of it in a week's time. He was threatening to leave her and get a divorce.

The Baileys and the Robinsons. Sandra Bailey came to the surgery to ask for a termination of pregnancy. She said her coil had fallen out and she was sure that she could not cope with another child. Her illiterate husband was many years older than her, and demanded a great deal of attention. They had a baby son who was often thrown around and never fed properly. They argued in bed about who should get up to attend to him.

The student had been to see Sandra's mother, Mrs Robinson, to learn about the background. Mrs Robinson had heart trouble and there had been several episodes of embolism. One of these had made her blind in one eye and partly paralysed her, but this had largely resolved. Her angina and asthmatic attacks prevented her from being as active as she wanted to be, so that she felt trapped. Her husband had once been in prison for stealing and when he came out he was obsessed with the idea of dying. Now he was back at work, but had become so worried by her illnesses that he was phoning her several times a day and became upset if she ever went out. He gave up all his other women.

At 60, Mrs Robinson was very much a matriarch. She had four children apart from Sandra: John, who had asthma and eczema and whose son had died from spina bifida; Denise, who had two daughters with asthma; Linda who had lost her son when he was a baby: she had taken him to the hospital because he was 'chesty' and was told not to be fussy. She had left her alcoholic husband the year before. Lastly, there was Fred and his wife, who lived with Mrs Robinson. After five years of anxiety and investigations, Fred's wife had become pregnant, but Mrs Robinson made it clear that she was going to take the baby over when it was born.

In discussing the issues raised for the doctors of the Riley and Robinson families three conclusions emerged:
1   It is often no more than a semantic quibble to call parts of a complex problem medical and parts social.
2   Which profession should do what is also likely to be a sterile issue. The roles of the doctor, the health visitor and the social worker are indicated less by formal definitions than by which of them is in the best position to help. They should keep in touch with each other and not stand too much on their professional dignity.
3   Knowing about a patient's social situation as well as his disease is useful, but the picture is not complete until his behaviour is considered.

REFERENCE SOURCES

Reid I. (1977) *Social Class Differences in Britain*. Open Books, London.
Brown G.W. & Harris T. (1978) *Social Origins of Depression*. Tavistock, London.

7. Psychological factors and psychological problems

It does not take long to observe that psychological problems are common, and that different doctors seem to find or attract them to a widely different extent. We can look at the difficulties posed by these problems under four headings: frequency, diagnosis, levels of complexity and effects on the doctor.

1 FREQUENCY

It is impossible to say objectively what proportion of consultations is concerned with psychological problems, because doctors differ in what they recognise. Such agreement as does exist suggests that the proportion is about one-third. Table 7.1 uses figures from a study of some general practitioners who tried to classify the psychological components in 553 consecutive consultations. Whether or not it is right to call them psychiatric is debatable.

Table 7.1 Frequency of physical and psychological components recognised in 553 consecutive consultations in general practice (Adapted from Goldberg and Blackwell.)

Doctor's assessment	% of patients	
Entirely psychiatric illness	7.8	
Psychiatric illness with somatic symptoms	9.4	
Psychiatric and physical illness, not related	5.4	32.7
Physical illness with associated psychiatric disturbance	1.8	
Physical illness in a neurotic personality	8.3	
Entirely physical illness		45.6
Other		21.3

2 DIAGNOSIS

Difficulties in diagnosis are caused by: lack of a satisfactory theor-

31

etical framework; imprecision in the diagnostic terms used; the interplay of psychological factors with physical, social and cultural aspects of the illness; and the need to establish connections between any psychological problems discovered and the presenting illness.

Lack of theoretical framework. With no good theory to guide them, general practitioners evolve pragmatic ways of dealing with problems related to the behaviour of their patients. Psychiatry has been of limited help, for as a speciality discipline it deals with a different range of conditions. The first group of diagnoses in Table 7.2 forms the bulk of the work of psychiatrists; conditions in the second group are very much more common in general practice but are not the main concern of any hospital speciality.

Table 7.2 Frequency in general practice consultations of two groups of conditions within ICD Category V, Mental Disorders

Diagnosis	% of consultations for Mental Disorders
Organic psychoses, schizophrenia, affective psychoses, paranoid states, other psychoses, phobic neurosis, obsessive compulsive neurosis, alcoholism and drug dependence	12
Anxiety neurosis, depressive neurosis, insomnia and physical disorders of psychogenic origin	72

NMS 2

Imprecise terminology. Psychiatric diagnostic terms are imprecise as used by psychiatrists, but in general practice the situation is even worse. Every general practitioner employs his own mixture of labels, culled from many schools of psychiatry and psychology and vague lay usages. 'Anxiety' and 'depression' are good examples of words which have no reliable meaning and are discussed a little later in this chapter.

Interplay with other aspects of illness. Possible relationships between the physical and psychological components of an illness were shown in Table 6.1. Pain, for example, is a very common presenting symptom of psychological disturbance, either as the direct result of muscle or gut tension, or indirectly when anxiety makes some minor painful condition intolerable. Psychological problems may be either the cause or an effect of social problems. An English doctor may not be able to distinguish between those reactions of a patient from another culture which are normal within that culture, and those which are peculiar to the individual.

Coexisting psychological problems. Just because a patient is found to have a psychological problem, it does not follow that this is the cause of his illness. Very few people have resolved all their psychological problems. To make this kind of illogical assumption is as slovenly as to conclude that an illness must have a psychological cause because no organic disease can be recognised. Positive reasons are necessary for psychological diagnosis too.

3 LEVEL OF COMPLEXITY

Psychological problems are not always very complicated at a practical level, and some can turn out to be quite simple.

A previously happy and healthy girl consulted the doctor complaining of tiredness and irritability, a month after the birth of her first baby. She wondered if she might be anaemic, which he thought unlikely, and then if the cause might be the pill—though she had been taking it for only a few days. When the doctor asked her how she liked being a mother, she 'froze' and seemed about to start crying. He told her that it was normal to swing between strong emotions, and that there was no need to worry if she felt hate at times. She stood up, held the baby at arm's length and said, 'I hate you' three times, then gave her a big cuddle. The 'illness' was cured immediately, and did not return.

Not many problems are as easily resolved as this one, and the doctor never knows what he is going to hear when he starts. Some will take many hours to understand or to treat, and concern about the amount of time involved is one reason for the reluctance of some general practitioners to begin. Other reasons might be: fear of being given a great deal of information which they will not know what to do with; fear that patients who are encouraged to talk will go on forever, getting more and more beyond the control of themselves or of the doctor; fear of having reactions that will affect their personal lives; and a feeling that there is no point in bringing things to light that may be incurable anyway. These fears often reflect inadequate training rather than psychopathology in the doctor.

4 EFFECTS ON THE DOCTOR

The diagnosis and treatment of every kind of illness takes place in the context of the relationship existing between a particular patient and a particular doctor. In a later chapter the influence of this context will be considered in more detail, but special problems may arise when the illness is primarily psychological. The very features of the patient's personality that are involved in the disturbance may be present in the doctor too (e.g. the story of Mrs F., p. 52).

ANXIETY AND DEPRESSION

Feelings of anxiety and depression are expressed in so many consultations and handled in so many ways that some confusion for students is inevitable. Some of the confusion is due to our ignorance about how the mind works, some is semantic, some is due to conflicting pressures on the general practitioner, and some to disagreement about methods of treatment.

SEMANTIC CONFUSION

A man relaxing over a brandy and cigar may say he is anxious about the future of western society; another man may say he feels anxious when he has to give an employee the sack. A woman may express anxiety about a lump found in one of her breasts; another woman may describe anxiety when she goes on a crowded bus.

Being depressed can mean being more or less unhappy, or feeling flat one day for no obvious reason; it can also be a lifelong personal trait, a paralysing reaction to loss or a sudden and inexplicable pathological state.

Until we are able to use the words more precisely, diagnosis and management will remain difficult.

PRESSURES ON THE DOCTOR

General practitioners are often told that they are too ready to ascribe everything to 'nerves' and to try to suppress normal feelings with drugs. They are also told that they ignore emotional problems and fail to recognise the desperate patient who is about to commit suicide. Faced with so many people who feel anxious and depressed, some doctors feel that more is expected of them than they have to give, and opt out in whatever ways leave them with the least guilt.

DISAGREEMENT ABOUT METHODS OF TREATMENT

The relative places of drugs, placebos, psychotherapy, behaviour therapy, physical treatments, reassurance, support, counselling and 'alternative' medicine seem to depend more on who is talking about them than upon the characteristics of the patients to be treated. Students are advised to be open minded but critical.

PRESENTATION

Patients may declare themselves to be anxious about something specific (which may or may not be medical, and may even be the very symptoms of anxiety, like palpitations or tension pains) or just generally anxious about everything. Anxious people may present with feelings of depression because they are tearful, exhausted, and frightened of the emotions they are experiencing. They may consult because of exacerbation of a duodenal ulcer or eczema; they may deny their anxiety, or fail to recognise its connection with their illness. Often there is a complicated mixture of physical, work, family and relationship problems. The doctor's recognition of the most tender areas, when he makes his verbal examination, may depend heavily on picking up non-verbal clues.

Depression may present with anxiety due to fear of morbid or obsessional thoughts or of terrifying and inexplicable feelings that are beyond control. It may present with a lack of energy and the feelings of failure that result, with loss of interest in food, hobbies, sex or people. It may be 'masked', the patient complaining only of abdominal pain or backache. It may be presented by a husband or wife, aware of changes in a spouse that are baffling or destructive. Again, non-verbal clues may be the most reliable guide in the early stages of a consultation.

When anxiety or depression is observed, its meanings and effects must be explored before anything else can be done; only then can a decision be reached on whether 'illness' can be diagnosed. To treat a normal reaction to a painful situation as an illness confuses and overextends the medical role, and while some non-medical roles are acceptable to some doctors (e.g. Counselling, p. 81), others are less so. To use drugs in such a situation makes the doctor a sort of barman—not an ignoble occupation but not a professional one either.

PSYCHOSEXUAL PROBLEMS

Everything that has been said about recognising, accepting, and coping with psychological problems applies with even greater force to problems that have a major sexual component. Sexual problems rarely, if ever, exist on their own, because sexuality is so fundamental that it has ramifications in every aspect of people's lives. Sexual problems are part of developmental, personality, relationship and emotional problems, and must be considered in context. Not all general practitioners are comfortable and competent in management, but recognition is inescapably part of their role.

Some idea of the ways in which psychosexual problems may present can be obtained from the following stories—five patients who were seen by one doctor in the course of one day.

A man of 42 who came for a repeat prescription of tablets for his epilepsy. After receiving it he revealed, with great difficulty, that he was having sexual fantasies about his four-year-old daughter and was terrified that he would assault her.

A man of 50 who asked for a small supply of diazepam: he used this when it was especially hard to stay off alcohol. Because he was a new patient he was asked about himself, and it became clear that there were problems in his marriage. Eventually he said that he was impotent with his wife but that he could sometimes just manage intercourse with a girlfriend. He asked for treatment so that it would be worthwhile leaving his wife and going to the other woman.

A woman of 48 who asked for some of the sleeping tablets she had been taking on and off for years. In the discussion which followed, and in subsequent consultations, she described how her husband had started to hate her twelve years earlier. He would deliberately excite her sexually and then turn over and go to sleep, a form of cruelty which she put up with for a year before divorcing him. Her previously normal feelings were so affected that when she remarried she constantly rejected her second husband sexually though he was both kind and considerate. Just when she began to think she might be able to to relax with him, he died of a sudden coronary thrombosis, leaving her with an enormous sense of guilt she could not resolve.

A man of 27 who reported a recurrence of pain from his prolapsed lumbosacral disc, which made it impossible for him to go to work. When asked, with deliberate ambiguity, if it caused any trouble in bed, he said he had not had intercourse for nearly a year because he was frightened he would provoke the pain. He had not been able to talk about this properly with his wife, and their relationship was deteriorating rapidly.

A boy of 15 who complained of a lump in the groin. No abnormality was found, but before getting dressed he asked, with apparent casualness, about a spot on his penis. When pushed fairly hard to reveal his real worry, he told how a woman friend of his mother had masturbated him and given him his only experience of fellatio.

None of these patients had committed themselves to talking about the sexual aspects of their problems when entering the consulting room, and the stories might never have come to light. On the other hand, the doctor must beware of seeming to pry into sexual matters when patients do not want to talk about them or regard them as irrelevant. Usually it is wise to proceed at a pace which produces only a small degree of discomfort.

Assumptions based on the doctor's beliefs about what is normal and what is abnormal are dangerous. It is safer to recognise that if anything can be imagined or done, someone has imagined it or done it; that anyone can feel guilty about anything; and that even people whom the doctor finds sexually repulsive have sexual feelings and sexual needs which they want him to understand.

THE FAMILY AND ILLNESS

Time spent in general practice provides an excellent opportunity to look at illness in a family context, and this means much more than seeing how families cope when one member is ill. The family can be observed defining illness and producing illness too.

DEFINING ILLNESS

Every society defines what it will regard as illness, and even a unit as small as the family has some influence in this respect. In one family, suffering from a cold may be totally ignored; in another, aspirins, lemon drinks or whisky may be offered even though the sufferer is expected to perform all his normal duties; while in a third, a visit to the doctor seems necessary. The definition may depend upon which member of the family has a cold. When symptoms are dramatic most families will react in the same way; it is when they are minor that a family tradition is most likely to make a difference. Serious illnesses sometimes start with minor symptoms, so acting in the family tradition may have important consequences.

PRODUCING ILLNESS

Tensions within the family can provoke symptoms which are taken to the doctor, and so can the problems which result when family beliefs and values collide with those of the world outside. The general practitioner needs to know who the members of a family are, and how it reached its present shape and size. For any further analysis, a list of some of the ways in which families can differ from each other is needed:

Roles. In every family there are roles that have to be taken— breadwinner, homemaker, peacemaker, and so on; ideally they are taken in a way that suits all the members. How satisfied each member is at any time is one way of describing a family. Another is the manner in which roles are altered when an illness or other change of circumstances makes this necessary. The alterations may be arrived at democratically or laid down by the most powerful member. Loss of role may be mourned as a kind of bereavement.

Patterns of interaction. There may be cooperation between all the members, conflict between all of them, or cooperating subgroupings in conflict with each other. The behaviour of one or more members may consist of little more than a reaction to the behaviour of another member. There may be intense involvement of pairs of members, e.g. husband and wife or mother and baby, so that the child or father feels excluded. Outsiders may be brought in as allies in family power struggles.

Authority. How authority is wielded, and where it lies, are important considerations, though not always easy for an outsider to determine. The amount of privacy—emotional and territorial—allowed to each member is a closely related issue.

Myths. It is not uncommon to find families in which everyone accords to one member an attribute which he does not possess and which at least some of them know perfectly well that he does not possess. 'Father makes the decisions in this house' and 'Jack's got more brains than the rest of us put together' are examples of such myths. At least one person derives a direct benefit from keeping the myth going, and it is rarely father or Jack in cases of this sort. Myths often centre around a presumed illness, where the potential for emotional blackmail is great; they are all the harder to fight against where the benefactor ascribes the illness to someone other than himself.

A woman may, for example, find that she can control her husband by insisting that 'Little Mary is very delicate' and therefore easily upset by his behaviour. To emphasise the point, the mother may take Mary to the doctor for a 'tonic' or something similar on occasion. If the doctor gives any kind of prescription or, worried by his inability to pinpoint the cause of the complaint, arranges investigations or a referral, the mother's hand is strengthened in her struggle with her husband. Ascribing illness in this way to a child is particularly nasty because the consequences may be far-reaching: Mary may well grow up believing that she really is delicate.

Themes. A degree of solidarity in a family is to be expected, but an unhealthy exaggeration is sometimes seen: 'We're a cut above the neighbours' is one variation, and leads to intense dependence of the members on each other. Conflict—with defeat for someone—is inevitable if, for example, a son wants to go out with the girl next door.

Atmosphere. The atmosphere in a family may be easier to feel than to pin down in words. Three of the key constituents are the balance of calmness and anxiety, the degree of restrictiveness or permissiveness, and the amount of emotional warmth. The atmosphere may be different for each child in a family because of the particular meaning he or she has for the parents.

COPING WITH ILLNESS

How a family copes with illness in a member depends to some extent on how the family defines it and on the part each member played in producing it. Roles must change—for the one who is ill, and for everyone else—with effects on the patterns of interaction, the location of authority and leadership, and perhaps on any myths or themes that may exist. A family may fragment under the strain, or grow closer together as it responds to the challenge.

The general practitioner is well placed to observe these reactions, and sometimes to modify them therapeutically.

DEALING WITH PSYCHOLOGICAL PROBLEMS

1 Psychological factors always need to be considered, if only to be sure that they do not constitute the illness.

2 The psychological effects of any intervention that the doctor wishes to make must also be considered.

3 The doctor needs both the inclination and the time, each of which may influence the other.

4 Skills in confrontation are required—an ability to face people with the effects of their behaviour on others, including the doctor. It is harmful for the doctor to ignore his own reactions until they erupt destructively. They can be used *diagnostically*, e.g. 'This woman makes me feel useless. If she makes her husband feel the same way, would this account for what is happening?' Hypotheses of this sort can then be explored, and the new, shared understanding used *therapeutically*.

5 The doctor has to recognise when he is not expected to do anything. Medical training stresses the importance of advising, investigating, referring and prescribing, so that doctors come to believe that professional care cannot be given without them. It is a great relief to discover that this is not necessarily true: some patients want no more than sympathetic recognition of how they are coping with insoluble problems; others want to see how the doctor reacts to fears and thoughts which are troubling them. A lack of activity is then reassuring and can help them bring these fears under control.

6 The doctor needs to use his imagination. This activity tends to be discouraged in students, which perhaps accounts for the mechanical approach to presenting symptoms and physical findings of which doctors are often accused. Good powers of imagination may be needed to fit together information from the records, from non-verbal cues and from the patient's answers; to find questions that make enough sense to a patient to encourage exploration of a painful subject; and to plan the sort of management most likely to be acceptable in each unique circumstance.

7 The doctor needs some insight into his own make up. If, for example, he still feels smothered by his own mother he will not be able to help a patient whose problem is similar.

8 The doctor needs a good referral technique. Suggesting that someone else should deal with a problem that has come to light is a delicate task if the patient is not to feel that he is being rejected. Sadly, the doctors least able or willing to deal with emotional problems themselves are likely to be the poorest in this respect too.

REFERENCE SOURCE

Goldberg D.P. & Blackwell B. (1970) Psychiatric illness in general practice. *Br. Med. J.* **2**, 439.

8. In the consultation

FACTORS IN THE INTERACTION

A social psychologist would analyse consultations in the same terms he might use for any meeting between two people. The more important variables could be:

The personalities of each: aggressive or timid, emotional or rational, etc.

The way each is feeling at the time: sad, anxious, angry, etc.

What each thinks of the setting in which they are meeting.

The uses to which each wants to put the meeting.

The significance each attaches to the meeting.

The view each has of the other.

The view that each thinks the other has of him.

What the first believes that the second imagines is the first's view of him—and vice versa.

What each actually says.

What each hears the other say.

What each thinks he is communicating non-verbally.

What each interprets by the other's non-verbal communications.

It is clear that there are many opportunities for misunderstandings to arise, and though no doctor will check every variable in every consultation, he does need to be aware quickly when a mismatch is occurring. In this chapter we will look briefly at the doctor, at why patients consult, at meaning and magic, at the uses and effects of the doctor-patient relationship and at ways in which this has been studied.

THE DOCTOR

Many sociologists have written about the medical profession and the difficulties that may arise because of the differences between the assumptions of doctors and patients. It is sadly true that one of the highest accolades patients bestow on a doctor is to say that he is 'really human'. There are two reasons for this: first, the doctor's social background is different from that of most of his patients—in terms of money, housing, schooling, expectations, life experiences, and use of language. Second, a medical education does more than provide a range of knowledge and skills. It gives a new vocabulary, and special ways of thinking about death, pain, illness, the body, drugs and the role of the doctor. It encompasses a host of beliefs that may fairly be called 'medical prejudices'.

The doctor is not usually aware of the effect of these differences, though he may sometimes wish that certain patients would think and behave more 'sensibly'!

WHY PATIENTS CONSULT

One of the consequences of being directly accessible to the public is that the general practitioner finds himself 'consulting' for many more kinds of reason than his training might have led him to expect. In the course of a typical day he will probably be consulted for all the following reasons:

1   For relief of symptoms, with or without a diagnosis.
2   For some other normal medical service.
3   For official recognition of sickness, e.g. certification.
4   For follow-up requested by the doctor himself.
5   For access to other parts of the health and welfare services.
6   For drugs on which the patient is dependent.
7   As an habitual response to anxieties.
8   To gain some psychological advantage in a relationship with others.
9   For support and recognition.
10 For playing games and acting out dramas.
11 For more than one of the above.

These reasons demonstrate that the doctor's role is not confined to practising medicine and fulfilling certain administrative tasks—it carries power which he and his patients use in many different ways.

MEANING AND MAGIC

In those consultations which *are* to do with illness presenting with symptoms, the traditional approach is to see the management as falling into two parts: first comes the diagnosis and then the treatment. The diagnosis is made by applying professional knowledge to the information which can be assembled from the doctor's memories about the patient, the medical records, answers to questions and a physical examination, supplemented by investigations or by talking to a member of the patient's family when necessary. Suitable treatment follows.

From the professional point of view this is fair enough, but it is a very doctor-centred way of thinking, whose limitations are especially important in general practice. For a worried patient the decision to consult is a major step, and the element of hope it contains is the true beginning of therapy.

The events which then take place before the consultation are important insofar as they affect this sense of hope—what other people say, the ease of making an appointment, the attitude of the receptionists, the ambience of the waiting-room and the time spent within it.

Even more important are the effects of many features of the consultation—what the doctor seems to know already, the effort he puts into trying to understand what the patient sees as wrong, how he asks his questions, the extent of his physical examination and how much care he appears to take over it, the look on his face as he makes it, and whether or not he decides to arrange any investigations. The history-taking, the examination and the ordering of blood-tests or X-rays are therefore part of the therapy. They may even be curative.

The phase that the doctor thinks of as treatment also needs to be seen through the patient's eyes. The advice, the exercises, the diet, the manipulation, the sick-note and the prescription have effects not only through their intrinsic scientific merits but also as they bear upon the hopes and fears in the patient's mind. To some extent, therefore, *treatments are interchangeable* and one may be as curative as another, which is why doctors may get equally good results using quite different methods. The prerequisites are that the doctor must seem convinced that his method will work, and that his decision to use it is thought to be based on a proper understanding of the problem. To say that histories or blood tests may be curative, or that any treatment may work if given with conviction and understanding, is not to suggest that medicine or general practice is based on magic. Most people who are ill are hoping to get better and the doctor's behaviour in either phase of the consultation should do nothing unwittingly to reduce this hope. In this light much of the magic has a perfectly rational explanation and nicely complements those aspects of treatment which are based on medical science.

EFFECTS AND USES OF THE DOCTOR-PATIENT RELATIONSHIP

The 'doctor-patient relationship' is a genuinely important subject, but discussions about it often lose contact with reality and are never constructive unless the terms of reference are clear. There are three separate perspectives which are liable to get confused, and each is beset with its own peculiar difficulties. The first is that of sociological role-theory, which tends to get abstract and ridden with jargon; the second is that of personal beliefs about the two roles which people debating the subject introduce—these form as poor a basis for a dialogue as sets of prejudices in any situation do; the third is concerned with analysing the way in which two specific people behave towards each other, when neither is likely to be objective about his own behaviour.

THE SOCIOLOGIST'S APPROACH

Sociological theories tend to fall into one of two main camps.

One starts with the proposition that everyone has certain social responsibilities which society expects him to fulfil, but that he may be excused them when he is sick. The status 'sick' has to be confirmed by an expert—the doctor—with whom the sick person must cooperate in order to get better and resume his normal duties as soon as possible. In return for this service to society, doctors are given certain privileges. The roles of doctor and patient therefore complement each other neatly, and the relationship is a harmonious one.

The second view is that doctors and patients must inevitably be in conflict. Patients' wishes and assumptions, and the meanings they give to symptoms, are bound to differ from those of doctors; the relationship of doctors and patients is inherently unbalanced because power is all on one side. Anyone who believes in complementarity and harmony is either very naive or else taking a doctor-centred view of the world.

A general practitioner might find some truth in both sets of propositions, but fail to recognise in either the truth about what goes on in his consulting room. Not every consultation is all harmony or all conflict, and power is not so unevenly distributed.

It is easy to see that many patients indeed start with wishes and assumptions different from those of the doctor, but most do reach agreement with him about what is to be treated and what has to be done. The process by which this agreement is reached is one of *negotiation*, conducted not by abstract 'role-bearers' but by real people, with the strengths and weaknesses of their individual personalities and beliefs.

PERSONAL BELIEFS

Every doctor has a view about his role and the nature of his relationship with patients in general. Four examples, simplified to the point of caricature perhaps, may be given:

a   The doctor is a wise parent figure, and patients are like children who have to be guided, praised, bribed or chastised to make them do what is good for them.

b   The doctor is a technical expert, adult and rational. Patients are also rational adults, quite capable of judging for themselves what is good for them.

c   The doctor is a mercenary of the NHS, and patients are the enemy. Each patient must be defeated, and any tactic is fair.

d   The doctor is a servant, and should be ready always to ignore his own convenience and convictions in fulfilling the expressed or unexpressed desires of his patients.

A rigid view of one's role is not a very helpful characteristic in general practice, though even the most idiosyncratic doctor over the years gathers to himself a clientele that likes his ways and is happy to complement them. This suggests that patient's beliefs fall into patterns similar to those of doctors and that reasonably well matching pairs are quite common.

RELATIONSHIPS BETWEEN PARTICULAR DOCTORS AND PARTICULAR PATIENTS

This level has immediate practical implications. How a patient relates to his doctor may decide when, where and how he presents his problems, the status he has in the negotiations, and the degree to which he complies with the doctor's management. How a doctor relates to a patient may determine how well he listens to the problem, the range of factors he takes into account, how he negotiates, how much trouble he takes, and how much he cares about follow-up.

It may also have long-term implications in the realm of the patient's attitudes to his own health and his responses to anything which threatens it. It is a very sensitive area. Exploring any relationship can be painful, and in this case the doctor is being invited to assess how much of his behaviour is governed by forces other than his professional knowledge and skills. The only justification for so threatening an invitation is that clinical decisions can have major effects on people's lives.

WAYS OF STUDYING THE RELATIONSHIP

One approach has been to look at the degree to which doctor and patient are active or passive. This is a rather limited way of looking at relationships, but it is worth considering. The idea came from the American sociologists Szasz and Hollender, who proposed three possibilities:
1 Doctor active, patient passive.
2 Doctor guides, patient cooperates.
3 Mutual participation.

The first of these would appear to be the most suitable in a medical crisis such as a major haemorrhage, the second in less serious acute illness, and the third in chronic illness, preventive medicine and various kinds of psychotherapy. The doctor should be capable of working in all three styles and of knowing when each is appropriate. It has been pointed out that there are other combinations within the model:
4 Doctor passive and patient active.
5 Mutual activity (but not in harmony).
6 Mutual passivity.
7 Patient guides, doctor cooperates.
   Each of these is seen on occasion.

Another approach is associated with the name of Michael Balint. He gathered groups of general practitioners who met regularly to talk as honestly as they could about patients who were causing them great difficulty. One of the purposes was for each doctor to learn what part his own behaviour was playing in creating the difficulty. Comparatively few general practitioners ever attended these seminars, but several books describing their work have been very influential.

A third approach has been to make audio or video tape recordings for later study. Just replaying them may have quite powerful effects, but several methods of analysing them in a structured way have also been devised. These make it possible to detect changes that take place over a period of time.

9. Eleven stories

This chapter consists of eleven stories, in each of which the intangible entity of 'relationship' had important consequences. The greater freedom of patients in general practice than of those in hospital makes it easier for the student to see the human element at work in medicine.

Miss A. was 35 and had made a mess of her life. She had held a number of jobs, usually as a shop assistant, and once as a nursing auxiliary. Her employers found her unreliable and inefficient, and she never kept any job for long. Eventually, her record made it impossible for her to get work, and she turned half-heartedly to prostitution. She had a little boy, and when he became old enough to be upset by the men who visited her, she gave up prostitution and lived only on Social Security. She had no friends and became increasingly withdrawn and depressed.

When she went one day to the surgery to ask for a cough medicine for her son, she was sent in to a general practitioner new to the practice. He asked her about her background, and because he had few patients to see he let her talk at length. He was impressed by her ability to tell a story and the shrewd insight of her observations about people; whenever he saw her after that he encouraged her to tell him more. He wanted to write a novel, and was looking for material, but after a while he realised that he could not use her experiences. He suggested that she should try to write a book herself, and, stirred by his interest and his belief that she could do it, she eventually started to write. The increase in her self-esteem made her a different person. The local newspaper printed a couple of articles by her, and she became friendly with some of her neighbours. Her book made slow progress and is unlikely to be finished. The general practitioner has not written his novel either.

It seems as though this patient's usual presenting symptoms were due to the poor opinion she had of herself, and that the doctor's personal interest in her helped to raise her self-esteem. In the next story, the unwitting effect of the doctor's way of behaving was to help his patient grow up.

Mr B. was in his middle twenties and had Crohn's disease. People tried not to get involved with him because he made scenes and threw tantrums if he was ever crossed. When it became clear that he needed major surgery and would be left with an ileostomy there was great apprehension about how he would cope with it. His general practitioner, a large and imperturbable man of 38, had never found Mr B. a problem. He had the knack of seeming unmoved by Mr B.'s outbursts, being helpful when they had some reasonable cause, and quite stern when they had not. Mr B. had never known anyone else behave like this with him, and always felt happier after seeing the doctor. He complained bitterly to everyone else about his illness and the need for an operation, but neither he nor his general practitioner had any doubts about his ability to manage an ileostomy.

If Miss A. and Mr B. found doctors with the right personal characteristics at the right time, the next five patients were not so lucky.

Mrs C., an old lady who lived alone, was very dependent on her general practitioner. He was 29 and had inherited the list of a retiring senior partner. There were many elderly patients, and he visited them all regularly and frequently—especially the old ladies who lived alone. He always sent them birthday cards, Christmas cards, and postcards when he went on holiday. Why he did this was not clear, but he certainly had a great need to be appreciated and loved, and perhaps it helped. Mrs C. thought he was marvellous, and when he suddenly left the practice she became depressed and her health deteriorated rapidly.

In satisfying his own needs, the doctor made his patient too dependent on him, and then let her down. In the next story the doctor had a need to get rid of a patient since his 'treatment' was affected by sexual feelings with which he could not cope.

Mrs D., a 30-year old divorcee, was admitted to hospital, having taken half a bottle of barbiturate sleeping capsules which she had obtained from her general practitioner. The story was as follows:

she had always been physically attractive, and, being aware of the powerful sexual effect that she had on men, she had never learned any other way of relating to them. Her general practitioner was a shy and serious man in his late forties; he had seen her twice in the month that she had been his patient. The first time that Mrs D. had consulted him, about a rash on her thigh, he had been uncomfortably aware of being aroused, but she kept things at a level that was no more than lightly coquettish and he was able to control himself without much difficulty. He looked forward to her next visit with mixed feelings.

When she came back a month later she seem very upset, but she calmed down after talking to him for a while. Her movements and appearance again aroused him, and when she leaned towards him, touched his knee and asked for 60 Sodium Amytal capsules, saying that she had needed them occasionally in the previous six years. He found himself unable to tell her he no longer prescribed barbiturates. His main wish was that she would leave, and the only way he could achieve this easily was to do as she asked. He gave her the prescription—though he ordered only 40 capsules. He felt very guilty when he learned about the overdose.

The remaining stories illustrate other ways in which a doctor may be 'wrong' for a particular patient.

Mrs E. was 27 and had a two-year-old child with spina bifida and paralysed legs. She came to her doctor quite frequently, not so much about the child as with her own complaints. These were principally: tiredness, headaches, dysuria, menorrhagia and vaginal discharge, in various combinations. She said that she got little help from her husband, and had no time to be ill because there was too much to do for the baby.

The general practitioner always sympathised with her difficult situation, and always supplied a prescription for the symptoms she presented. From occasional remarks made by Mrs E. he had some idea that all was not well in her marriage, but this was never discussed. He was a man who found it difficult to talk about sexual and marital problems, and his own marriage was under strain at the time. He did not know Mr E., who was a patient of another practice. An unspoken agreement developed between the doctor and Mrs E. not to mention what was going on in her marriage, but he gave her his time generously and treated all her symptoms assiduously. He was very surprised when her husband left her, but he did offer to give her antidepressants!

Mrs F., a woman of 50, consulted her general practitioner, a woman of the same age, about a painful shoulder, though it quickly became clear that this was not very important. She was travelling a total of three hours every day to look after her mother, a fit 75-year-old, who was quite capable of looking after herself. Mrs F. said she was made to feel unbearably guilty if she tried to protest at her mother's demands.

Because the general practitioner had a similar, though less severe, problem with her own mother, she felt both sympathetic and useless. Telling Mrs F. to be firm did not sound very convincing to either of them. She could think of no real way to help, and ended the consultation by prescribing two aspirins four-hourly for the presenting complaint. Five days later Mrs F. was admitted to hospital because of a haematemesis.

These two patients were unlucky to have doctors with unresolved problems similar to their own, and who could respond only by 'medicalising' the presenting symptoms. In one case the drug treatment was a collusion to avoid facing the real problem; in the other, the irrelevant symptomatic treatment did active harm.

Colonel G. had been invalided out of the army in his late forties after a head injury which left him suffering from epileptiform attacks. He was on anti-convulsants which he obtained from his general practitioner. Usually he sent requests for his prescriptions by post, and it was obvious from the intervals between requests that he was not taking the tablets as instructed. Occasionally he came to the surgery in person; the general practitioner would then try to clarify the discrepancy and find out about Colonel G.'s alcohol consumption. He always failed because he felt intimidated. The Colonel spoke loudly, ignored questions when it suited him to do so, made the doctor feel socially inept as well as professionally impotent, and always walked out as soon as he had his prescription. The general practitioner had never been good at coping with aggressive men, and had no way of dealing with the Colonel.

One day Colonel G. had a violent fit while being driven by his wife, causing her to go off the road and into a tree. Both were quite seriously injured.

This was a patient any doctor might have found difficult, save perhaps one who behaved like a general. It should be remembered that patients sometimes pick doctors for their weaknesses.

These seven stories raise serious questions. Must it always be the workings of chance, or someone's self-destructive urges, that determine whether a doctor's personality brings benefit or harm to a patient? What is the doctor's responsibility? He cannot make himself perfect for every situation, but is there a point at which his professional competence becomes an issue? The next few stories suggest ways in which he may come to modify his behaviour.

Mr H. was 19 years old when he left home, came to London and signed on with a new general practitioner. He told his doctor that his father had been ridiculously strict with him and that there had been a serious row before they parted. Mr H. was an epileptic on sodium valproate tablets which he said he was supposed to take three times daily. The general practitioner told him earnestly that he must take them as directed. A week later, in the evening, the general practitioner was called to Mr H.'s bedsitter because of a grand mal attack that was over by the time he arrived. This happened twice more in the next fortnight, making the general practitioner pretty annoyed. After the third attack he firmly laid down the law, saying that Mr H. was old enough to know better and that the tablets were for his own good. If he did not take them properly in future he would have to find another doctor.

Watching the young man's face the general practitioner was suddenly aware that this was a scene which Mr H. knew well. He stopped in mid-sentence and after a pause said, 'Oh Lord, I'm behaving just like your father.' Mr H. said nothing and the doctor left. The next visit for a prescription was made at the right time. The patient smiled, but made no reference to the earlier events; the general practitioner smiled and forbore to give any instructions. An unspoken bargain must have been struck, because there was no trouble after that.

This case history illustrates the use of empathy. The doctor suddenly saw himself through his patient's eyes, and changed his approach accordingly.

Whenever *Mrs I.* consulted her general practitioner he found himself promising to do things for her. When she told him about her older son's difficulties at school he rang the headmaster and the Director of Education. He wrote several long letters to the Housing Manager and made three phone calls to the Social Services Department about her house. When she was dissatisfied with a surgeon who found no cause for alarm in a prominent vein on her younger son's penis, he made an appointment with a different surgeon. In short, the general practitioner always saw things in her terms, and sympathetically took up the cudgels on her behalf. Mrs I. rarely thanked him for his efforts—she would be too full of her latest problem—but he told himself that he should not expect gratitude just for doing his job, and this made him more vulnerable to the next complaint. In fact, she never actually asked him to do anything; he offered because he reckoned that he would be able to do more for her than she could do for herself.

Mrs I. rarely mentioned her husband, though once she indicated that he was 'pretty useless', and that in the previous five years they had had intercourse only three times. One day she said that she was trying to improve the marriage, and that it would be easier to do this if her husband's hours of work were changed. She wanted the general practitioner to phone the personnel manager at her husband's firm to see if this could be arranged. For obvious reasons, she said, she did not want her husband to know that this was being done behind his back. The general practitioner felt that this was going too far, and protested. She began to cry and said that her marriage would certainly break down. To temporise, he promised that he would think about it, but the more he did so in the next week, the more angry he felt with himself for always rushing to her 'rescue' in the past. He was honest enough to recognise that he should not take this anger out on Mrs I., but he wondered how he would react if she got angry with him for not doing what she wanted.

At the next consultation she asked him if he had made the call. He gave her a conspiratorial grin and said, 'You know what to do, don't you?'. She seemed to understand this cryptic remark and did not raise the subject again; in fact, she ceased trying to manipulate him from then on. Indirectly, he learned that her marriage did improve, and he often wondered if his relaxed refusal had come at a critical moment when she really was frightened that her husband would leave her.

For a long time the doctor had been satisfying needs of his own in a way that brought short-term advantages to a manipulative patient. He changed when he saw his previous actions in a new light; with luck the shock might make him review his behaviour with other patients to whose 'rescue' he had been accustomed to ride.

A third possibility for change in the doctor arises if he uses his feelings about a patient diagnostically.

Mrs J., a widow of 60, had more complaints than even her general practitioner believed possible. At each visit she produced between four and eight, and none was described in any textbook of medicine. In the course of just over a year he had given her four kinds of sleeping tablet, four different analgesics, four tranquillisers, two antidepressants, two laxatives, two rubefacient creams, two 'tonics', an anticholinergic, and a cholagogue. Not only did these fail to make her better—they usually made her worse, as she told the general practitioner more in anger than in sorrow. His inability to satisfy her made him feel impotent and frustrated, and he wished very strongly that she would leave him alone. He kept on because he was conscientious, but he would get rid of her as soon as he could, pushing a prescription into her hand and leading her to the door.

One day, when her complaints seemed even more directed at him than usual, he felt anger welling up inside him. Instead of shouting at her or pushing her out as usual, he said as calmly as he could that she was beginning to make him angry. The result was dramatic: she stopped, and in a small voice said that everyone was angry with her. The general practitioner's anger vanished. Suddenly he felt concern for her; he felt that at last she had given him somewhere genuine to start from. She went on to say that her daughter and daughter-in-law were both avoiding her. She felt lonely and terrified of being deserted, but her fear came out as aggressiveness, and she was driving everyone away. With a little encouragement she thought of a few ways in which she might act differently, and later she tried them out. She made several more visits, in which she was more hopeful and self-critical; the general practitioner felt more useful and no longer pushed her out with a prescription. After a month she stopped making appointments.

The general practitioner was so impressed by the effects of being honest that he resolved to adopt the same policy with other patients who were a problem to him. After several further successes he thought he had found a panacea, until an experience with Mr K. taught him some caution.

Mr K. was a 50-year-old foreman with a chronic duodenal ulcer. He never took any notice of the advice his general practitioner gave him about his diet, his smoking, or his way of living, and he never completed any course of treatment. Instead, he preferred to take large doses of magnesium trisilicate with belladonna mixture, sometimes very frequently.

He and his wife lived next door to his mother, and both women were well known to the general practitioner. Mrs K. junior was a pale, thin woman who took sleeping tablets every night and lived in a state of quiet desperation. Mrs K. senior was a large, hypertensive woman, left partly disabled by a stroke. Mr K. usually slept in his mother's house, and often spent the whole evening there. He played his wife and mother off against each other, leaving them both unhappy and insecure. The general practitioner discerned a clear pattern in Mr K.'s behaviour. With his wife, his doctor, and his mother he wanted everything on his own terms, not caring about the effects of what he did as long as he remained in control. At his next visit Mr K. announced that he had been very upset by someone at work who had called him a selfish bastard and hit him. The general practitioner saw his chance to apply his new policy of honesty.

He replied that perhaps this episode deserved some thought. He too had occasionally felt like hitting Mr K., and perhaps at times both Mr K.'s wife and mother might have had the same desire. Did Mr K. understand why people should feel that way? Mr K. became very abusive and left the consulting room muttering threats. He complained to the Family Practitioner Committee that the general practitioner had been negligent in the treatment of his mother, and added his suspicions that the general practitioner was having an affair with his wife. It was nearly a year before the Disciplinary Service Committee finally dismissed the charges, a very unpleasant time both for the doctor and others involved.

It was probable that the doctor's feelings led him to a correct and justified interpretation of Mr K.'s behaviour, but at that point he stopped thinking. Mr K. was deriving such advantages from his selfishness and was so upset by the man who called him selfish and hit him, that he was most unlikely to respond to an invitation to rational self-appraisal. It was as if the doctor had diagnosed tonsillitis and automatically prescribed penicillin without stopping to ask about penicillin allergy.

From the first seven stories it is apparent that the doctor-patient relationship has clinical effects. From the last four it is clear that studying this relationship can make a doctor more clinically effective.

10. Home visits

Visiting patients at home is an important feature of the work of general practitioners. In most practices, house calls now account for about 15-20% of all consultations or, in other words, several every working day. Most of them are made on a round, at about the same time each day. The round includes new calls, 'repeat' or follow-up calls, and some regular visiting—usually of the elderly.

There can be no doubt of the popularity of house calls with the general public, but the number made has steadily declined over the last 20 years. Reasons offered for this decline include: a higher proportion of patients with cars, greater difficulties caused to doctors by traffic congestion and parking problems, a reduction in the number of bed-ridden patients, changes in medical attitudes towards rest in bed, and an improvement in clinical and nursing facilities in the practice premises which has led to the view that consultations there, rather than at home, use the available time more efficiently.

General practitioners tend to have mixed feelings about home visits. On the one hand, it is satisfying to diagnose and treat serious illness or cope with emergencies using a minimum of equipment, and the appreciation by an elderly invalid of a regular visit is certainly heartwarming. On the other hand, unnecessary calls, perhaps at awkward hours, engender quite different feelings. About a half of British general practitioners make regular use of commercial deputising services for out-of-hours calls; most of the rest work some kind of rota with their partners or with other practices. The reduction in home visits has been welcome to general practitioners, but it is rare to find a doctor who wishes to do away with them altogether. They are seen as having some real value other than the personal satisfaction that they bring and the economies that accrue to the NHS when illness is treated at home rather than in hospital. The value lies in the way that they may assist both diagnosis and management.

The degree of cleanliness, tidiness and affluence of homes and gardens, and the ways in which members of the household behave towards each other, all offer information which the general practitioner may need either immediately or in the future. The context of his work is that of a continuing relationship, so the more he understands about his patients the more efficient he can become in diagnosis, management and prognosis. When he has seen them in their homes, patients are more likely to feel that he knows them better and to believe that his advice will be relevant. For many people relationships are more satisfactory when they have an opportunity to give as well as to take and they welcome the role of host.

Home visiting also gives the doctor a chance to function preventively: to observe likely causes of accidents, to see the need for a handrail or a repositioned electric socket, to judge the temperature at the time or as it might be when the weather is colder, or to comment on the danger of a loose staircarpet. Though some calls are requested for trivial or inconsiderate reasons, much serious and chronic handicapping illness is seen at home—one measure of this is the much greater proportion of consultations in the home which result in hospital admission. The likelihood of these kinds of illness is higher in elderly patients, and calls to the elderly are more frequent than to other age groups.

Whether general practitioners should visit their elderly patients regularly rather than only upon request is a contentious subject. Such visiting is usually (though not always) appreciated, but there is an inherent danger of the visit becoming no more than a social call, with matters of medical importance being missed. One solution is for some regular visits to be made by the health visitor and some by the doctor. Information from a recent large survey of people aged 65 and over illustrates the present situation. The percentage of the elderly that had been visited in a six month period by certain 'officials' from the health and social services and voluntary organisations is shown in Table 10.1. The insurance man was included in the list because he is known to go to many homes. Many people over 65 are, of course, active and do not require visits, but the figures do suggest that some changes might be valuable. 30% of elderly people live alone—over three-quarters of them are women, and over a third are women aged 75 or more.

Visits during terminal illness must also be mentioned. About 23 patients die annually in the 'average' practice, and while only

Table 10.1 Percentages of the elderly receiving visits from selected 'officials' by type of household (A. Hunt, 1978)

Visits received from:	Total %	Live alone %	Live with others %
Doctor	33.3	28.4	35.5
Health visitor	4.4	5.6	3.8
District nurse	7.8	7.6	7.9
Home help	8.9	18.9	4.0
Council welfare officer	3.9	5.9	3.0
Social security/supplementary benefits visiting officer	6.0	9.0	4.7
Meals on wheels	2.6	6.4	1.0
Mobile library	2.8	2.8	2.9
Other official person	3.6	3.8	3.4
Voluntary organisation	2.7	2.8	2.6
Minister of religion	16.2	17.6	15.6
Insurance man	48.7	36.5	53.8
None of these	25.0	28.5	23.5
Insurance man is the only visitor	23.4	17.0	26.2

a quarter of them die at home, many of those who die in hospital spend part of their last illness at home. A great deal is demanded of the general practitioner, in terms of medical skills, empathy and commitment, to help the patient have a good death, and the relatives an uncomplicated bereavement.

REFERENCE SOURCE

Hunt A. (1978) *The Elderly at Home.* HMSO, London.

III. The resources available

Introduction

The general practitioner has many resources available to him in dealing with the clinical problems he faces. They are described in the next four chapters.

Even in a short attachment to a teaching practice it is likely that several examples from each category will be seen in use. Because resources tend to differ from one place to another, the list of facilities under each category cannot be exhaustive.

11. Resources: the patient, his family, and friends

Each general practitioner has about 1500 beds (some single, some double) and a very large number of people available to assist in looking after his patients. His reliance on the help of patients and relatives is enormous, though it may be neither fully acknowledged nor tapped.

The doctor does not always hear how patients have endured pain, tried to help themselves or tolerated medical inefficiency rather than complain. He is more likely to be aware of the few who are over-dependent. Relatives and others often rearrange and disrupt their lives to help someone who is sick, providing much of the necessary nursing and psychological support. In some instances, help with more technical procedures is sought: a spouse is asked to record the partner's sleeping pulse rate, or a woman to take her temperature on waking as part of investigations for infertility. Patients with diabetes test their urine, fill in charts, and inject insulin—even estimate serial blood sugars with a reflectance meter. Other equipment loaned for use at home includes mini-flowmeters, sphygmomanometers, relaxation audiocassettes, and incontinence alarm kits. Physiotherapy has been taught to patients for a long time—e.g. tipping for people with bronchiectasis—and many physiotherapists believe that, because their time is so limited, the only way they can treat more people at home is to teach them what to do and then supervise their efforts intermittently. Finally, every general practitioner can quote a story of some patient or relative who has devised an ingenious apparatus to assist treatment in the home.

Perhaps doctors are too conservative. There seems to be no good reason why people other than diabetics should not learn to give injections—in pernicious anaemia or painful terminal illness for example. Greater willingness by the doctor to treat people as partners in fighting disease and adversity might liberate a creative energy that would enlarge his resources.

63

12. Resources: within the practice

There is considerable variation in the premises, the equipment, and the people who work in practices.

PREMISES

The most important difference is that between health centres and other kinds of surgeries. It lies in who owns the building. Whereas most surgeries belong to, or are leased by, the doctors who work there, health centres are owned by the NHS, and the doctors pay a rental to practise from them. There may be any number of doctors in either kind of premises, though the average in health centres is over five and in other surgeries about three.

There are at present about 1250 health centres in the UK and roughly 6500 general practitioners—a quarter of the total—work from them. Staff employed by the District Health Authority of the NHS—nurses, health visitors and midwives—may be attached to any practice, though they are less likely to be found outside health centres.

Services like speech therapy, audiology, community physiotherapy, chiropody, and school dentistry are traditionally provided in special clinics, but are likely to be based in health centres where these exist.

EQUIPMENT

In addition to the basic medical tools, practices may own diagnostic equipment such as ECG machines, peak-flow meters and microscopes, and administrative equipment such as dictaphones, photocopiers, radiopaging machines and computers. The level of equipment, however, will be found to vary greatly.

THE RECORDS

From everything that has been said about the interview, it is clear that recording it succinctly is liable to be difficult. There is much current debate about records in general practice, the details of which are not directly important to the undergraduate. The debate is about the purpose of the records: whether they are primarily an aide-memoire for the doctor who makes them, or should be a more structured and complete display of data intended to be easily assimilated by other medical and non-medical members of the primary care group.

There are those who believe that using bigger paper would be enough—the present small folder was designed over 60 years ago. With or without bigger paper, others would add summary cards, family sheets, and flow charts; some prefer to separate the different problems of a patient under special headings; and a few would have everything arranged so that it can easily be coded for computer storage. The importance of recording in preventive medicine is discussed in Chapter 17.

At the very least the records should be legible and chronologically ordered, with the important positive and negative findings easily seen. This state of affairs is far from being universally attained as yet, but it is becoming obligatory in practices that wish to be involved in vocational training.

PEOPLE

The kinds of people who work in practices, or 'primary health groups' are becoming more numerous and more varied. There are established general practitioners, trainee practitioners, and people employed by the doctors like secretaries, receptionists and practice nurses. Very often there are staff attached by the DHA—nurses, health visitors and midwives. More rarely there are geriatric visitors from the DHA, social workers from the local authority, counsellors from the Marriage Guidance Council, or dieticians, psychologists, physiotherapists and others who arrive from a variety of sources. It is fashionable to call the whole group a 'team', but this can be misleading, since some of the members are independent of the doctor and have their own professional objectives.

OTHER DOCTORS

Only about one general practitioner in seven now practises single-handed, and the proportion continues to decrease. The last bastion of solo practice is the inner city, especially in London. In the last 30 years groups have been getting larger, and some contain more than twelve doctors. The average is nearly four.

Some degree of specialisation has emerged: one partner may do most of the obstetrics, run a child development clinic, or fit the caps and coils for the practice. Unusual skills, like manipulating spines or syringing tear ducts may be made use of by the other doctors, and partners frequently seek each others' opinions over coffee. On the other hand, the idea of structuring a practice around formal areas of specialisation—one doctor for the children, one for the elderly and so on—is unpopular because it ignores and threatens the basic values of general practice. The special skill of the general practitioner lies in recognising the nature and complexities of the problems presented to him and making basic decisions about them, rather than in a detailed understanding of pathological processes; nor is there great need of the latter when a specialist's opinion is readily available on referral.

NURSES

Nurses employed by general practitioners are called practice nurses, and work mainly on the surgery premises. They usually have rooms of their own and do whatever they and the doctors agree to be within their competence. They dress wounds, give injections, syringe ears, test urines and take blood, and in many practices they now test vision and hearing, record ECGs, and do work of a much less traditional kind. The number of practice nurses is growing and is currently about 3500.

District nurses are employed by the DHA, and most of them are attached to general practices. They see the patients of the practice and do much of their nursing in the patients' houses. The work that they may perform is governed locally by the nursing hierarchy and is undertaken by SRNs, SENs and bath attendants, according to its complexity. District nurses have a long history of working with general practitioners to make treatment at home and early discharge from hospital possible. There is an increasing trend for nurses

employed by the DHA to work in treatment rooms in doctors' surgeries, especially in health centres.

HEALTH VISITORS

Health visitors are employed by the DHA and most of them are
attached to practices. The health visitor's training is long—she must
be a registered nurse and a midwife before spending a year studying
human development, the family, some educational psychology,
social aspects of health, and social policy, to obtain her certificate.
Her work has five main aspects:
1 The prevention of mental, physical and emotional ill health, and
its consequences.
2 Early detection of ill health and the surveillance of high-risk
groups.
3 Recognition and identification of need, and mobilisation of
appropriate resources where necessary.
4 Health teaching.
5 Provision of care. This includes support during periods of stress,
and advice and guidance in cases of illness as well as in the care and
management of children. The health visitor is not, however, actively
involved in technical nursing procedures.

Much of this job specification is rather intangible in nature, and
a great deal depends on her personality.

Health visitors are involved mainly with pre-school children,
partly in their homes and partly in clinics in the surgery. The most
important feature to note is that, unlike the district nurse, she has
access to patients independently of her relationship with the general
practitioner. She discovers problems about which he might not
otherwise have known, just as he finds problems to refer to her.
This useful symbiosis has come about since the policy of attachment
began, and it is still quite new. For many practices the health visitor
has become the natural link with the Social Services department of
the local authority.

MIDWIVES

Community midwives are employed by the DHA and often attached
to practices. Their role in home confinements has all but disappeared.
They share antenatal care and postnatal visiting in various ways

with general practitioners and, in some places, both of them attend the confinements of practice patients in maternity units—which may be within a hospital, associated with a specialist unit.

COMMUNITY PSYCHIATRIC NURSES

Community psychiatric nursing is a comparatively new development and the nurses are still based mainly in hospital departments of psychiatry. Some work both in hospital and in the community; very few are attached to general practice-based primary care. Most of their patients are referred to them by psychiatrists.

They visit patients in their homes to monitor progress, give long-acting phenothiazine injections, and offer support or sometimes psychotherapy or counselling. Close collaboration with the patients' general practitioners is needed, and in some districts good relationships have grown up. Difficulties arise because of problems over clinical responsibility: since the patients are at home this lies with their general practitioners, but when they have been referred to hospital-based nurses by hospital-based psychiatrists it may not be clear that this is so. The way forward would seem to be for the service to become part of community nursing.

RECEPTIONISTS AND SECRETARIES

The receptionist's job can be the most difficult in the surgery. She is expected to work efficiently under pressure both from doctors and patients. Her value may extend well beyond her formal role, since over many years she will have learned a great deal about the patients, the doctors, the locality, and whom to contact about what.

A secretary may have similar virtues and be a similar resource. In some practices the senior receptionist or secretary is called a practice manager or administrator, doing most of the administrative work and much else besides.

PATIENT PARTICIPATION GROUPS

In a small but growing proportion of practices (under 1%) patient participation groups have been created. Their suggestions may produce changes in the way that a practice is organised, and they sometimes run support groups, transport services or collect prescriptions.

13. Resources: hospitals and other medical agencies

INVESTIGATIONS

General practitioners have direct access to the district X-ray and pathology services which are based in hospitals, and about 11% of the work of these services is at their request. Some hospitals also provide an ECG service.

There are great differences between general practitioners in the frequency with which they ask for investigations, and in the range of investigations called for. National figures for 1980 suggest that a general practitioner with a list of 2000 patients requested, on average, about 450 pathology tests and 1300 X-rays. Some of the factors associated with frequent use are: being young, working in a group, having a middle-class practice, and being within easy reach of the services. The ways in which specimens reach the laboratory vary greatly, and so does the speed with which the results are returned. It has been noted in studies of investigations ordered by general practitioners that they are more likely to show some abnormality than those requested within the hospital. This probably reflects the general practitioner's tendency to use them to confirm a diagnosis rather than as a routine procedure.

DIRECT ADMISSION

A general practitioner with an 'average' list will send about one patient a week into hospital as an emergency—though another four will also be admitted via the Casualty Department, from waiting lists and following domiciliary consultations arranged with consultants. Admissions are made for social as well as medical reasons. They are much more common for elderly patients, and the rate is higher in rural than in urban areas. In some places, especially in the winter, admission may be difficult to arrange and waste a great deal of the general practitioner's time. General practitioners sometimes visit their patients in hospital—probably most commonly in small towns where there is only one hospital.

Patients usually welcome such visits, which can also be used for an exchange of information and ideas between the general practitioner and hospital staff. A system that encouraged the general practitioner to remain involved with his patients in hospital might be beneficial to everyone concerned.

Community hospitals, in which the general practitioner looks after his own patients who need admission but not the resources of a general hospital. There are more than 400 of them in the UK and about 4000 practitioners use them. They are distributed unevenly: in south-west England they account for almost a third of the medical beds, but in north-west London only one-twentieth.

OUTPATIENT REFERRAL

The general practitioner with an 'average' list refers about six patients a week to outpatient departments, though again the variations are considerable. Referral rates are highest in London. Many people also attend Casualty Departments, often without being referred.

Outpatient services generate many of the complaints that general practitioners and hospital doctors make about each other. Hospital doctors complain about the inadequacy of the information they receive and about evidence of lack of clinical interest on the general practitioner's part. General practitioners complain about the long waiting lists, delays in reports, failure to have specific questions answered, and the unwillingness of some clinics to discharge a patient.

EDUCATIONAL

Roughly a quarter of all general practitioners assist in the work of a hospital department, and this service can be important educationally. In addition, library facilities, especially where there is a postgraduate centre, are usually available to general practitioners. Many consultants contribute to the continuing education of general practitioners by way of ward rounds, demonstrations and lectures.

MISCELLANEOUS

The obstetric flying squad; the coronary care ambulance.
Day hospitals—especially for psychiatric patients.
Direct access to dieticians, physiotherapists and others, in some hospitals.
Domiciliary visits to patients in their homes made by consultants on request.
Hospices, for the care of people who are dying.

NHS RESOURCES OUTSIDE THE HOSPITAL

The ambulance service.
Clinics for family planning, cervical cytology, chiropody and various preventive child health services—often housed within Health Centres, where these exist.
Health Education Officers.
The Public Health Laboratory Service.
Poisons information centres.
Community based physiotherapy in a few places.
Emergency Bed Bureaux.
Information—journals and circulars from DHSS.

THE PRIVATE SECTOR

Private medicine, outside London, assumes major significance only for abortion services, where a large proportion of the work is done by non-profit-making organisations.
Emergency deputising services, which are used by about 45% of general practitioners.

14. Resources: non-medical agencies

There is often confusion between Social Security, which is a service of central government, and the Social Services department of the local authority. Social Security provides:

Non-contributory benefits, e.g. child benefit, family income supplement, supplementary benefit, attendance allowances, mobility allowance, and industrial injury benefits.

Contributory benefits, e.g. maternity, sickness, invalidity, unemployment, death grants.

Certain services for those who qualify, e.g. relief from prescription charges, dental charges, and charges for glasses; reimbursement of fares to visit hospitals; free school meals, milk and vitamins; rent and rate rebates, and legal advice. It is at the Social Security Office that the Disablement Resettlement Officer can be contacted to help a disabled patient find suitable employment or training for a new job at a special centre.

DEPARTMENT OF SOCIAL SERVICES

This is a part of local government at the level of the county council or metropolitan district (the boroughs, in London). It provides a huge range of daytime, residential and domiciliary services for children, the elderly, the homeless, and the physically and mentally disabled. It is also responsible for social services within hospitals. Its functions are summarised in Table. 14.1.

Social services reach the public mainly through teams of social workers in the community, and many of a general practitioner's patients will be clients or potential clients of social workers. From the general practitioner's point of view some of the main reasons for contacting the Social Services for his patients are: to get a home help, to obtain meals-on-wheels; to gain access to a day centre or luncheon club; to have alterations made to homes or get gadgets

72

Table 14.1 Functions of a Social Services Department

---

1 Research into social needs.
2 Evaluation and development of the services provided.
3 Extending public awareness of the services provided.
4 Providing domiciliary care, protection and supervision for those in need:
especially children, the disabled, the elderly and mentally disordered (who may need to be committed to hospital). This heading also covers home helps and ancillary services.
5 Providing day centres for those in need:
including day nurseries, 'intermediate treatment' centres for children, workshops for the disabled, and training, occupational and social centres for the mentally disordered and the sick and infirm.
6 Providing residential care, hostels and holiday homes for a wide range of people in need:
including temporary accommodation for those with nowhere else to go.
7 Other miscellaneous services:
including registering adoption societies, children's homes and child minders, homes for the disabled and the elderly, charities for the disabled, and homes for the mentally disordered. The department also acts as an adoption agency and a guardian *ad litem*; it produces reports for the courts in care proceedings, manages the property of those in care or in hospital and provides for the burial or cremation of those for whom no suitable alternative arrangements are available.

---

and appliances for the disabled; to find a place in a day nursery; to have a patient admitted compulsorily to a mental hospital to prevent possible non-accidental injury to a child; and to gain information about other agencies providing money or help (including Social Security). In addition, he may also wish to make use of the social worker's skills in case work, which may be defined broadly as working with people to help them learn how best to help themselves in their current difficulties.

General practitioners complain that social workers are too woolly minded, take too long to get anything done, cannot maintain confidentiality because of their organisational structure, and move around too frequently to provide long-term support. Social workers complain that doctors have only the vaguest idea of what they do and of the difficulties that they face, generally adopt an authoritarian approach very different from the ethos of social work, and are too ready to resort to medication. Many doctors find it hard to regard social work as an independent profession, with its own knowledge, skills, values, prejudices and difficulties; and, though this situation should improve as time goes by, it may be for the good of the public that some tension between the two professions should remain, based on genuine differences of approach.

In a few places social workers have been attached to general practices, becoming part of primary care groups and dealing with the population of the practice. This has created an opportunity to improve understanding and communication not just between social workers and doctors, but also between social workers and health visitors, nurses, midwives and other members of the group.

OTHER ORGANISATIONS

The general practitioner's knowledge of his locality and of people in it are a major practical resource.

Locally, the general practitioner will get to know chemists, opticians, dentists, vets, the police, ministers of religion, head teachers, the coroner's officer, MPs, members of the local authority, industrial personnel officers, Citizens Advice Bureaux, the Samaritans, the Community Relations Council, the WRVS, dieting clubs, 'good neighbour' associations, refuges for battered wives, Church Army and Salvation Army hostels, Rotary and Round Table, and a host of other organisations and people.

There is an enormous variety of associations and charitable trusts providing housing, nursing, holidays, meeting places, advice and practical help for people with particular diseases, disabilities and disadvantages. No general practitioner or health visitor could hope to remember them all; they tend to rely on the experience and contacts of the social worker to produce the best answer.

Finally, general practitioners might with advantage keep informed about what is on sale in local sex shops.

IV. Some specific skills

Introduction

It is not expected that a student should learn the particular set of skills that is required in general practice, but he should know what they are. He may require them himself or expect them of colleagues in the future.

Since the consultation has a function which is different from that of a hospital specialist, the interviewing skills required are different. The causes and effects of the difference are explained, and special attention is given to the difficulties which students experience in the interviews they conduct themselves.

In recent years there has been a growing recognition of the need for a preventive approach to illness. More attention is given within the consultation to diet, exercise, smoking and drinking; many special clinics have been organised, often involving health visitors; practices have begun to audit the effectiveness of their work, and to think in epidemiological terms of the needs of the patient-population as a whole. These developments are reflected in skills required of the general practitioner, and two chapters in this section outline what is involved.

15. Interviewing

There are, in general, two kinds of interview: those held for the benefit of the interviewer—prospective employers or interrogators, for example—and those conducted for the benefit of the person being interviewed. Medical interviews should exemplify the latter.

Different kinds of medical interviews have different purposes, and the purposes determine their nature. The interview in general practice is inevitably different from the interview in hospital, for four reasons.

1 The specialist is trying to discover if his highly concentrated knowledge and skills can be of help to the patient. The general practitioner's patients have not been medically sorted; he can therefore make no assumptions about what kind of illness, if any, may be present. Nor can he make any assumptions about what patients' symptoms mean to them. Making unwarranted assumptions is a major potential hazard for the general practitioner; these may be psychological, social and cultural, or medical.

Psychological. The doctor does not try to find out what the patient thinks and feels because:
a He believes he knows.
b He takes it for granted that the patient will have the same reactions as he does himself.
c Trying to find out might be embarrassing.

Social and cultural. This is a poorly defined area in which the doctor can easily go wrong. It includes such matters as use of language, socially shaped attitudes to work, education, authority and the family, and attitudes more specific to the patient's family of origin and place of work. The doctor's belief and values may not hold true in the patient's world.

77

Illness, symptoms, doctors and treatments may have meanings to someone of another culture that the doctor would not even consider, while poor English may compound the problem.

Medical. The doctor may mistakenly assume:

a That the body-system of the presenting symptom is a good clue to the kind of illness that is present, e.g. that a vaginal discharge must mean gynaecological pathology.

b That patients always want consultations to keep to the normal medical model of diagnosis followed by treatment.

c That patients make the same kinds of association between various clinical phenomena as doctors do, even if less expertly.

d That what the patient presents is independent of his relationship with the doctor.

It would be unrealistic to expect that every assumption should be checked at every consultation—surgeries would never finish. There are times, however, when more care than usual is needed:

With new patients.

When the patient's culture is unfamiliar.

When there is a situation with a high emotional charge.

When the doctor becomes aware of unexpected resistance to 'sensible' advice.

The doctor's power and status may be harmful if they reduce his awareness of the assumptions he is making, but they also make it possible for him to ask the highly personal questions needed to avoid these assumptions.

2 The second reason for the differences in interviewing arises from the different morbidity in the two settings. The range of illnesses seen is virtually identical—any illness may be seen in either—but the probabilities are very different. The tables in Chapter 1 make the point clearly.

Probability underlies the approach of all clinicians—*no* doctor takes a complete history or performs a complete examination. In the hospital specialties there is a high probability that the doctors will be most efficient if they develop a special kind of history taking and examination appropriate to their discipline. In general practice there is a high probability that it would be a waste of time to explore an illness to the point of exact diagnosis when it bears the hallmark of being minor and self-limiting. History taking, examination and investigation in general practice should not be judged by standards derived from another setting. Nevertheless, the student will find the process of diagnosis in general practice pretty familiar, and his stock of knowledge reasonably useful.

3 The third difference comes from the general practitioner's knowledge about his patients, stored partly in his head and partly in his records. He may see an individual not only with different illnesses, but also in a variety of different roles and situations. He will, then, know his patients—and they know him—in ways which are unavailable to other kinds of doctor.

He does not know all his patients so well: they may not consult him, or they may be new to his list; he may be unperceptive or forgetful. When this is the case, his interviewing becomes more like that of a hospital doctor in some respects.

4 The final major difference is that of the time perspective. All doctors use time diagnostically and therapeutically, being gratefully aware that with its passing many things become clearer and that much is healed. The distinguishing feature of general practice is a perspective that relates to the very short-term and the very long-term. The general practitioner sees numerous brief illnesses, few of which will have direct significance for the years ahead. He also deals with the impact of chronic disabilities on people's lives, and long-term patterns of health and ill health. A continuing relationship implies that nothing is ever truly finished, and no consultation is complete and self-contained. Every interview affects the next one, and is affected by the previous one. Because he is easily accessible to his patients, it is not too fanciful to think of his contact with a patient as one interview extended over many years.

These four differences—the greater importance of avoiding assumptions, the morbidity, prior knowledge about the patients, and the time perspective—have practical consequences for the interview.

a More time must be spent finding out what the consultation means to the patient, and organising undifferentiated complaints into some kind of pattern.

b Less time need be spent on learning about the patient's past history and social history.

c In the early part of the interview, the doctor's questions may need to be very open ended, so that the patient can direct him to the problem area. 'Does the pain go down the back of your thigh?' is a good question only when there is no doubt that the pain is what should be discussed. 'Tell me about the pain' may be answered in terms of the patient's memories of his father's illness, of complaints about a supervisor at work, or of sexual problems, leading in directions the doctor would never have predicted.

d   Non-verbal cues become an important source of information in the phase of determining what the interview is about.

e   Again, in this early phase, the doctor may use his own reactions to the patient diagnostically. Feelings of depression may mean that the patient is depressed; feelings of anger may give the clue that the patient makes other people angry, and so on.

f   Some of the information the doctor may need is easily obtained from other members of the patient's family, and it helps if the doctor knows something of the dynamics of the families he sees.

g   The doctor may choose to do a little of the work at a time, and make frequent follow-up appointments.

h   Unless he wants a patient to leave his list, the doctor will try to avoid actions that strain their relationship. At times he may have no choice but to accept statements he doubts, or give prescriptions and certificates difficult to justify objectively, in the hope that he is preventing the breakdown of a relationship which may in time become clinically useful.

i   The doctor has to take into account his patient's psychological make-up and social situation as well as his physical state when he plans to make any intervention, just as he has to when making his overall diagnosis. The treatment of pneumonia involves more than giving antibiotics—the patient is kept off work and put into bed; and sterlising people is not just a matter of tying their tubes.

j   The doctor's view of a situation does not always go unopposed. There is frequently a period of 'negotiation' over what is to be treated, and how.

The list on p. 43 indicated that medical and bureaucratic problems were not the only reasons for consulting a doctor. Two activities that need special mention are support and counselling.

SUPPORT

Some patients have to live with problems for which there is no solution, and value the emotional support that their general practitioner can give them. For this they need his tacit agreement that they may come to him every so often and tell him how difficult things are. He need do no more than show sympathetic recognition of their problems. Every general practitioner has patients like this, and fills an important need in their lives.

Reaching the stage where this happens easily can sometimes be difficult: the patient's complaints about his life may be interpreted as 'complaints' in a more medical sense. Prescriptions, investigations and even referrals follow; and the inevitable failure of these actions makes the doctor feel useless and frustrated. Sadly, he may come to dislike the patient.

Sympathy is a powerful weapon, not to be confused with pity, which may be resented, or with friendliness or courtesy. The effect of sympathy is to encourage people to keep going in their present way, and it is therefore appropriate when the aim is to support. It is not appropriate when an unhappy situation could be improved if the patient stopped feeling sorry for himself and did something positive. The indications for sympathy need to be clearly understood.

COUNSELLING

This is a grossly misused term, too often applied vaguely to any situation where the 'helping' person spends more time talking than usual. This is a pity, because it has a proper meaning and a proper place.

It is *not* a treatment or therapy—even a psychotherapy—and it is therefore not appropriate for anyone diagnosed as emotionally ill. It is applicable in situations where people are finding difficulty in making up their mind what to do, for reasons that they do not understand, and who therefore may be experiencing symptoms of anxiety. The counsellor asks them to talk about this difficulty, essentially doing no more than ask, 'Why?', 'How?' or 'Can you explain that more clearly?' at crucial points, until the person being counselled becomes clearer in his mind what the real problem is and what he wants to do about it. At no stage does the counsellor offer insights, suggestions, or advice. This is a more difficult task than it sounds, and may not often be appropriate in general practice. Calling other activities counselling, however valuable and helpful they may be, leads only to confusion.

NOTES FOR STUDENTS
INTERVIEWING PATIENTS

A consultation needs both substance and shape. The substance consists of what is known about the patient, and the gathering of adequate information depends on a number of skills. The shape is imposed in the course of the interview, and learning to set the priorities and aims which determine it is far more difficult than mastering the skills.

THE SKILLS

These are listed below under three headings. The first group consists of normal courtesies which should be extended to every patient. The second contains some skills which will be needed in almost every interview; not all of them come naturally to everybody. These basic skills, together with the normal courtesies, allow the patient to communicate everything that he wants to communicate. The advanced skills are used to take things further—they push against resistances or help the patient understand matters which he did not understand before.

Normal courtesies
1 Introducing oneself and making sure one knows the patient's name.
2 Paying attention—especially not gazing around, writing or interrupting when the patient is trying to explain something, or looking too casual.
3 Letting the patient express his ideas without being disparaging or defensive.
4 Showing warmth.
5 Avoiding language that the patient does not understand.
6 Not jumping to conclusions.
7 Making sure at the end that the patient understands what is to happen next.

Basic skills
1 Using open-ended questions, especially in the early stages.
2 Encouraging the patient to talk by allowing some silences, following the leads he gives rather than sticking to a list of questions,

and, when he stops in doubt, repeating his last few words with an interrogative inflection.

3 Indicating understanding by occasional summaries of what has been said so far, so that the patient knows it is safe to move on.

4 Encouraging the patient to show how his mind is working by probing his ideas and by reflecting some of his questions back at him (e.g. 'What should I do?', 'What do you reckon your options are?').

5 Drawing testable inferences from the major non-verbal clues (style of dress, kemptness, body movements and the contexts in which they occur).

6 Deciding what should be achieved by the end of the interview.

Advanced skills
1 Using the patient's ideas constructively.
2 Using one's own feelings diagnostically.
3 Using silence.
4 Offering interpretations.
5 Confronting, without being aggressive or rejecting.
6 Touching the patient.
7 Changing the direction of the interview when it is leading nowhere.

SHAPING THE CONSULTATION

As soon as the student forsakes the safety of the systematic questioning he learned at an earlier stage, he is exposed to the danger of the shapeless interview. This is a situation in which the patient passes on his confusion rather than his information, the student loses his bearings, and each hopes desperately that the other will find an acceptable way out of the circular conversation in which they have become trapped. It can be avoided.

In every consultation there is a moment, usually in the first five minutes, when its main features are recognisable. Much information may still be needed to define the issues clearly, but the student can see at least *what kind* of problems he has to deal with. At this point he should review everything relevant that he knows and set himself one or more realistic goals. It is often helpful to discuss them with the patient.

It is a misconception to believe that the interview is not complete until all the patient's problems have been laid bare and solved.

Some situations are best not thought of as 'problems to be solved'; not all problems are soluble; some are too complex for one interview; many need intermissions in which both parties have time for reflection. There is no law that says how many appointments will be needed or how they should be spaced. A realistic goal is one whose achievement makes the patient want to keep his next appointment.

The following list of 'shapes' is not exhaustive, but it covers most of the possibilities that the student will meet.

1 The problem is simple and straightforward; the goal can be to deal with it there and then.

2 The problem is too big for one session, or there are several problems. The aim is to agree with the patient what will be dealt with and what postponed. Sometimes the problem first presented can be safely ignored.

3 The patient wants something other than a medical diagnosis and treatment: information, explanation, a sympathetic ear or help in making a decision. This may not be easy to recognise but the immediate goal will usually be to provide what is wanted. The student may consider that the patient's wants differ from his needs, so that other goals are discernible.

4 The patient's emotional state makes it impossible to discuss his problems—he is too angry, too anxious or too withdrawn, for example. The immediate goal must be to cope with this, even if it means that the underlying problem remains temporarily unexplored. At times the emotional state is so extreme that it *is* the diagnosis, so that the goal becomes immediate appropriate action.

5 Patient and student have very different views on what the symptoms mean or on what should be done about them. The goal is to negotiate some common ground or strike a bargain. If this proves impossible the consultation should be terminated, but the first concession may have to come from the student.

6 The patient is avoiding something which is likely to be important. The goal is to get him to understand the effects of doing this in such a way that he is able to consider changing his mind, perhaps at the next consultation.

7 The patient is not being straight—he is trying to manipulate the student, furthering a myth or simply lying. The goal is to express this calmly and to indicate firmly that there is no point in carrying on with the consultation in these circumstances.

8 The patient, who has hitherto bottled up his emotions, has reached the point where everything comes tumbling out. The aim is to indicate non-verbally that this is acceptable and should not make the patient feel ashamed. An intermission is sometimes necessary before the revelations can be used constructively.

Classifications of this sort mean something only at a very general level. Each consultation has a shape of its own, determined by the needs and interaction of those taking part in it. To say that there should be a shape means no more than that doctor and patient should each feel that they have got somewhere and that their time has not been wasted.

16. Defining the needs of a practice population

NEEDS

'Needs' is a difficult word, and in the shifting triangle of forces formed by social expectations, economic reality, and the beliefs of the professions involved, they can be placed at any point which satisfies the speaker's prejudices. Health Service planners at district, regional and national levels study their populations and try to decide how 'needs' can best be satisfied with the resources available. General practitioners are to some extent involved in such planning because of their local knowledge, as members of District Health Planning Terms.

A practice population may be quite different from even a district population—the patients of two practices in the same district may not have similar 'needs'. A practice population as such is not likely to be of interest to anyone except the general practitioners concerned, and those who work with them; but the patients of the practice may be considerably affected by the ways in which it organises itself to meet their 'needs'.

INFORMATION

Ideally, the organisation of a practice should be based on a great deal of accurate information about its population of patients—total numbers, age-structure, birth rate, mobility, social class structure, employment, the prevalence of chronic illnesses and incidence of various acute illnesses—and about the medical and social services in the area. Every general practitioner is informed about the size of his list, and how many of his patients are over 65 and over 75 by the Family Practitioner Committee that bases part of his income on these facts. Any further information about his practice he must find for himself.

Even without it he will know that he has, for example, many young couples, largely in semi-skilled and unskilled occupations, living on housing estates, and with a high birth rate; that there are a great many older men with chronic bronchitis; that in winter he finds it hard to get patients into hospital; that the social services are pretty patchy; that surgeries are busier than they used to be, but house calls are getting fewer. These impressions would not satisfy professional planners, but they will shape the way that he organises his work and his ideas about whom he wants to have working with him.

Many general practitioners do gather information, believing that it will enable them to be more efficient, and even to offer services designed to reduce future 'needs'. The three basic ways are:

1 Counting the number of consultations. This may be done differentially for surgery attendances and home visits, for morning and evening surgeries, for new and follow-up appointments, and for the various members of the group. The information may be used as it stands, or in conjunction with subjective impressions, to reorganise or redistribute work.

2 An age-sex register of the practice patients can be constructed. Any high-risk group that can be defined in terms of these two variables can be identified if the practice wishes to adopt some preventive measures for the members. Used in conjunction with work load figures it may be possible to see where extra resources are needed.

3 A disease index showing which patients have consulted with certain diseases; some kinds of index also show how often these patients consult.

Other activities that, in theory at least, are easy to monitor are prescribing, repeat prescribing, and how often certain items of service like immunisation, cervical smears and contraceptive advice are undertaken.

Setting up such information systems is not easy, but the knowledge gleaned from them may be important to others besides the doctor—nurses and, particularly, health visitors may be able to plan their work more efficiently as a result. It is possible that the production of hard data may persuade a health authority or local authority to deploy its services differently.

A few practices have even more elaborate information systems, using computers. Such systems are difficult to introduce into group practices because they cannot be sustained if they require more effort than the least-motivated member of the practice is willing to make.

If changes are made on the basis of information gathered, the next step is to measure the effects of the changes. This is operational research. Clinical research can be based on the same tools, modified if necessary. The scope for this is increasingly being recognised, and more practices are becoming interested in individual or co-operative studies. The defined population of the practice list allows some kinds of research that would be impossible in countries with a different system of primary care.

17. Education and prevention

The general practitioner's role in educating his patients and preventing illness is undertaken partly in the normal process of consulting and partly by way of special arrangements.

IN NORMAL CONSULTATIONS

All clinical consultations have educational or preventive aspects. As the following examples show, patients learn not only from explicit advice, but also both directly and indirectly from the questions they are asked and from what the doctor does.

EXPLICIT ADVICE

'Part of your back trouble is due to the way you lift things. I'll show you a better way.'

DIRECT LEARNING FROM THE DOCTOR'S QUESTIONS

'When I saw you about the rash on my hands I remember you asked if I was coming into contact with anything different, and I said I wasn't. I forgot I'd been staying at my mother's, and she has a different kind of washing powder. Could it be that?'

DIRECT LEARNING FROM THE DOCTOR'S ACTIONS

'I didn't realise that wax could make you so deaf till you syringed my ears.'

INDIRECT LEARNING FROM THE DOCTOR'S QUESTIONS

People learn what interests a particular doctor by the sort of ques-

tions he asks: for example, whether he tends to avoid or to emphasise psychological aspects of a problem. They learn how to be a
patient for each of the doctors they consult.

INDIRECT LEARNING FROM THE DOCTOR'S ACTIONS

Consider the different long-term implications of:
a 'That's a nasty cough. I'm giving you an antibiotic to make sure
it doesn't go to your chest.'
b 'Here's some medicine for your cough. I want you to take it
regularly every four hours.'
c 'I can't cure your cough. It should be gone in a week anyway but
I'll give you something to soothe it in the meantime.'
d 'It's just a cough. It'll be gone in a week whether you buy your-
self a cough medicine or not.'

It is almost impossible to imagine a consultation with no educational or preventative implications, and because general practitioners have continuing and fairly close relationships with their
patients, what they teach and what they prevent is important.

SPECIAL ARRANGEMENTS

In the past, general practice has been organised mainly to react to
whatever presented itself. There is now a belief, held fervently by
some, that a less passive approach is necessary: illness should be
prevented if possible or, at least, detected in its early, presympto-
matic, stages. The closer connection of general practitioners with
health visitors, whose work is based on a philosophy of education
and prevention, has fostered this change. Modern methods of practice organisation make it easier to implement, though much remains
to be done.

The special arrangements that can be made may first be considered in terms of activities with the *well* and with *high-risk groups*.

THE WELL

The commonest activities are:

Well baby clinics. Babies are examined at this type of clinic for
conditions such as deafness, congenital heart disease and dislocation of the hip; assessed in their physical, intellectual and

emotional development; and immunised against a number of infections. A very important additional benefit is the chance that mothers get to talk to each other.

Well woman clinics. These clinics are concerned mainly with examining breasts and taking cervical smears.

Contraceptive clinics. These may be combined with the well woman clinics. Alternatively, contraception may be dealt with in normal surgery sessions. A few practices perform their own vasectomies.

HIGH-RISK GROUPS

The only activity commonly separated from normal consulting sessions is antenatal care. Clinics are often held in cooperation with an attached midwife or health visitor. The practice may be taking full responsibility for a patient's antenatal care, or sharing it with a specialist unit.

Some practices systematically assess the problems of their elderly patients, in cooperation with health visitors, geriatricians or both.

Special clinics may be set up to help patients stop smoking or lose weight, as an alternative to supervision in normal surgery sessions. The same may be done for people with conditions needing regular monitoring such as diabetes and hypertension.

The recently bereaved are another high-risk group, though surveillance is more likely to be made in normal surgery sessions—often on the pretext of some other health problem.

Picking up hypertension is one of the most important screening activities possible in general practice. In some surgeries the blood pressure of all patients in a specified age band (say 35-55) is measured, whatever the reason for consultation.

Discussion and advice for people about to retire from work may prevent problems later on. In some practices, especially health centres, groups are run for them and for the retired.

Other kinds· of patients' groups, encouraging self-help, have been started in a few places, but little is known about them yet.

SCREENING AND EARLY DIAGNOSIS

So far, the subject has been considered in terms of activities which

Chapter 17

the student is likely to see. In considering the needs of the future, a more theoretical approach is required.

The idea of detecting diseases in their very earliest stages, before they cause symptoms, is an attractive one, and a great deal of thought has gone into considering the circumstances in which it is ethically, scientifically, and financially justifiable to try to do this.

The following principles are generally agreed:

1   The condition being sought should be an important health problem for the community.

2   The natural history of the condition should include a recognisable latent, or early symptomatic, stage.

3   There should be a procedure acceptable to the population which can detect the condition in this latent, or early symptomatic, stage.

4   Early treatment of the condition should favourably influence its course and prognosis.

5   There should be an agreed policy on whom to test.

6   Facilities should be available for the diagnosis and treatment of people who show a positive result to the procedure.

7   There should be an acceptable form of treatment for patients in whom the condition is diagnosed.

8   The whole cost of the endeavour (which includes the cost of diagnosis and treatment in those with a positive test) must be socially acceptable in the context of the cost of medical care as a whole.

9   Detection should be a continuing process, rather than a once and for all project.

DEFINITIONS

Preventive medicine utilises a number of terms which, if used loosely, can create confusion. The following definitions should be observed:

Screening. The 'presumptive identification of unrecognised disease or defect by the application of tests, examinations or other procedures which can be applied rapidly'. These procedures try to sort out, among apparently well people, those who have the disease or defect from those who probably do not. They are not intended to be diagnostic, so that a person with positive findings needs further consideration before a diagnosis can be made. Screening procedures may also be used to identify people with known risk factors, like high blood pressure or abnormal blood lipids, as well as those likely to have unrecognised disease.

When screening is carried out on the whole population, or on a major sub-group such as all adults, the programme is known as *mass screening*. When it is applied only to sub-groups known to be at high risk because of age, sex, occupation etc., it is called *selective screening*. Programmes that include many different kinds of procedure are described as *multiphasic screening*.

Case finding. This is the use of *diagnostic* procedures, with no clinical indications, on a group of people known to be at special risk, so that the disease may be diagnosed and treatment offered.

Validity. Since screening procedures are not diagnostic, the investigator needs to know how 'good' the ones he is using are. The validity of a procedure is the frequency with which the results obtained by using it are later confirmed by diagnostic test. It may produce both false-positive and false-negative findings.

Sensitivity. The ability of a test to give a positive result when the person really does have the disease.

Specificity. The ability of a test to give a negative result when the person does not have the disease.

It is possible to make a test so specific that there are no false positives, but this will eventually be at the expense of its sensitivity. Alternatively, a test can be so sensitive that there are no false negatives, though at the expense of its specificity. In practice, some compromise is usually accepted.

METHODS IN GENERAL PRACTICE

Since each general practitioner has a registered list of patients, it would be possible for him, using an age-sex register, to undertake true screening of the whole of this population or some major sub-group of it. In the face of the criteria mentioned earlier, and the effort involved, this very rarely happens.

There are two alternatives. The first is to run regularly various clinics which appropriate people are encouraged to attend—the well baby and well woman clinics mentioned above being good examples. The second is to use the contact provided by ordinary consultations. The general practitioner sees about 90% of his patients over a period of three years, and can therefore perform the tests in which he is interested on most members of the target groups when they attend for other reasons—checking the blood pressure of anyone aged 35-55 is a good example of this approach. These two alternatives are more easily sustained than special population-based projects and they make use of one of the fundamental strengths of general practice—the element of continuity. They also pose problems.

Where there is continuity of care it should be possible to detect some illnesses at an early stage by recognising change over time in certain variables such as biochemical tests, ECG tracings or, perhaps, even behaviour patterns. This suggests a need both for baseline data about each patient and for a recording system from which information can be retrieved easily. Despite the pioneering work of many individuals there is as yet no implemented agreement on what data should be routinely recorded, when they should be recorded, or about whom they should be recorded. Nor can most practices retrieve information easily. These are tasks that must be tackled if general practice is to fulfil its potential for detecting illness in its early stages.

REFERENCE SOURCES

Lancet (1974) A series of papers on screening published between October and December 1974.

Commission on Chronic Illness (1957) *Chronic Illness in the United States Vol 1.* Harvard University Press, Cambridge, Mass.

V. Conclusions

18. The functions of the general practitioner

The student will see the general practitioner serve such a confusing variety of functions that the following analysis may be helpful.

He provides primary medical care. Most people go first to their general practitioner when they are ill, and even when they are away from home they can sign on as a Temporary Resident with another practice. Much preventive medicine is part of primary medical care. Cooperation with the district community health service has led to the concept of *primary health care*, and this is increasingly practice-based. Other important functions of primary medical care include: referring patients to specialist services when necessary; issuing a variety of statutory and non-statutory certificates; and directing patients to non-medical agencies which may be able to help them.

He provides personal and continuing medical care. More than 60% of people have been registered with their general practitioner for more than ten years or since birth. The continuing relationship has many advantages: he is in a position to coordinate their medical care; he learns things that make the diagnosis and management of their illnesses easier; the organisation of preventive measures is facilitated; he can develop a personal influence which makes him a particularly effective educator; and he has opportunities for research which are lacking almost everywhere else in the world.

Access to the general practitioner is simple, non-stigmatising and free, and his social status is high. The result of this unique combination of circumstances and functions is that his patients present him with a wide range of problems. His first, and often his most important, task is therefore to understand why a patient is consulting him. This is sometimes extremely difficult. Mistakes may have serious consequences for his patients and incompetence could result in overloading of the hospital services to the point of collapse. The general practitioner is the only kind of doctor trained to take this responsibility; defining the nature of undifferentiated problems

into differentiated problems

is therefore his primary skill. Until he has exercised it he cannot bring any of his other skills to bear.

For problems he defines as non-medical he may suggest the help of a suitable expert, but sometimes he will cope with them himself:

1 He may give advice, making it clear that his opinion is personal, not expert.

2 He may undertake counselling if he is trained in the requisite skills.

3 He may give emotional support, at which his medical status rather than his medical knowledge may make him particularly effective.

For medical problems he may believe that the patient needs information, explanation, advice or reassurance rather than diagnosis and treatment; and different skills are demanded by each of these activities.

One other function must be mentioned—medical teaching. One general practitioner in ten is an approved vocational trainer and a quarter of all practices are training practices. In addition, many hundreds of practices are involved in undergraduate teaching.

Educate   At Every Consultative

Aim of consultati

Present problem / preventive

Other problems / health

modify health

seeking behaviour

19. Considering the future

One aspect of working in general practice has not yet been mentioned: the chance given to the student of assessing it as a possible choice for his own future career. A rational assessment depends not only upon the features found attractive, but also upon the extent to which present deficiencies can be put right. General practice has changed in so many ways in the last 20 years that predictions are risky, but the expectations of today's undergraduates will be one of the forces bringing change about.

It seems safe to foresee continuing development of medical technology. General practice will gain more efficient and reliable means of diagnosing and treating patients outside hospitals; and the more elaborate technology of hospital specialties and sub-specialties will probably increase the need of the public for a personal doctor who can bridge the gap between undifferentiated complaints and the latest marvels of science. None of the general practitioner's current roles is likely to disappear, though all may be modified.

Putting right deficiencies in the application of existing knowledge and services will surely remain the biggest task, particularly in relation to the elderly, who will constitute an increasing proportion of the population for some years to come. General practice must conduct its own research, absorb scientific advances, improve its information systems, cooperate with other branches of medicine and other professions, and stay flexible enough to reorganise itself to meet public needs.

The principles which underlie these tasks should become apparent to the student: they are important for him to understand whether or not he decides to enter general practice. The choice of career that he makes will be an informed one if he has seen the intense involvement a good general practitioner feels for work he finds fascinating, and has become aware of the effort that is being put into defining and providing an appropriate postgraduate training.